Health Services and Health Hazards:
The Employee's Need to Know

WITH CONTRIBUTIONS BY

Frank C. Abbott
New York State Education Department

Robert L. Biblo
Harvard Community Health Plan

Paul N. Bloom, Ph.D.
University of Maryland

John D. Blum, J.D.
Boston University Center for Industry
and Health Care

Joseph Boffa, D.M.D.
Boston University School of Graduate
Dentistry

George R. Dunlop, M.D.
American College of Surgeons

John Friedland
Boston University Center for Industry
and Health Care

Donald R. Giller
Boston University Medical Center

Emlyn I. Griffith
New York State Board of Regents

Bruce W. Karrh, M.D.
E. I. DuPont de Nemours

H. Cranston Lawton
Aetna Life and Casualty

Kenneth J. Linde
Department of Health, Education, and
Welfare

Robert S. Lurie
Harvard Community Health Plan

Barry Rabner
Boston University School of Graduate
Dentistry

Robert D. Reinecke, M.D.
Albany Medical College

Ronald Stiff, Ph.D.
University of Baltimore

Linda Kay Stokes, J.D.
InterStudy

George B. Strumpf
Department of Health, Education, and
Welfare

Diana Chapman Walsh
Boston University Center for Industry
and Health Care

INDUSTRY AND HEALTH CARE 4

Health Services
and Health Hazards:
The Employee's
Need to Know

Edited by
Richard H. Egdahl and
Diana Chapman Walsh

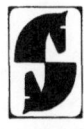
Springer-Verlag New York

Springer Series on Industry and Health Care
Richard H. Egdahl, M.D., Ph.D.
Diana Chapman Walsh, M.S.
Center for Industry and Health Care
Boston University Health Policy Institute
53 Bay State Road
Boston, Massachusetts 02215

Springer-Verlag New York Inc.
175 Fifth Avenue
New York, New York 10010

Health services and health hazards.

(Springer series on industry and health care; no. 4)
Based on discussions and background papers associated with a conference held in
Boston, Nov. 4–5, 1977.
Includes bibliographical references.
1. Medical care—Information services—United States—Congresses. 2. Labor
and laboring classes—United States—Congresses. 3. Advertising—Medicine—
United States—Congress. 4. Medical care—United States—Marketing—Congresses.
5. Health maintenance organizations—United States—Congresses. 6. Industrial
hygiene—Information services—United States—Congresses. I. Walsh, Diana Chapman.
II. Egdahl, Richard Harrison. [DNLM: 1. Industrial medicine—United States—
Congresses. 2. Occupational health services—Congresses. WA412 H434]
RA395.A3H427   362.1'07   78-18241

9 8 7 6 5 4 3 2 1

ISBN-13: 978-0-387-90335-4   e-ISBN-13: 978-1-4612-9948-6
DOI: 10.1007/978-1-4612-9948-6

Preface

Close followers of the evolution of the Series on Industry and Health Care will recognize in this fourth volume some continuity and some change. The essential concept behind the series remains: here, as before, we are looking to private industry as a potential agent of change in the American health care delivery system. We have made some structural accommodations, however, to comments received from readers in industry and in health services.

The original concept of a topical monograph supplemented by a separate hardbound volume of background papers has yielded to the present formula in which each volume is complete in itself. The series continues to draw much of its material from interdisciplinary working conferences convened by the Boston University Center for Industry and Health Care. Rather than publish conference proceedings, we have again undertaken to analyze the discussions and to integrate with them some timely background materials. Readers have found this format a major improvement over traditional conference reports and summaries.

Future volumes are planned on a range of topics: the effectiveness of prepaid health plans (HMOs) in containing health care costs; the role of insurance carriers in designing, administering, and monitoring employee benefit programs; occupational stress and corporate mental health programs; hormone rhythms as related to work, sleep, stress, and travel. To make the series as useful as possible, we are alert for possible new topics and we solicit suggestions from readers on questions they would like to see explored. Because each volume is planned, written, and produced in under a year's time, the series affords the opportunity for unusually rapid turnaround on subjects of strong current interest.

The conference undergirding this volume, held November 4–5, 1977, in Boston, was entitled "Employee and Employer Decisions About Health: Informational Issues." Eighteen background papers were circulated to participants in advance; the conference itself consisted of a lively give-and-take without formal presentations. Thirteen of those papers, edited and significantly condensed to conserve space, appear as part II of this volume.

We are grateful to the contributors of those eighteen papers, and to the remaining conference participants for sharing their expertise with us. And we owe several additional debts of gratitude.

Willis B. Goldbeck and the Washington Business Group on Health have provided guidance, advice, and information essential to the development of the series generally and to the preparation of this volume. William J. Bicknell, M.D., was, as usual, incisive and extremely helpful in his critical review of the manuscript.

With extraordinary competence and good humor, Susan Kelleher and Antonette Doherty attended to the many administrative, technical, and logistical details involved in assembling the pieces of the book and securing the necessary clearances from contributors and quoted conference participants. Susan Kelleher also helped with the early library research.

Into Janet Marantz's capable hands fell the difficult task of substantially reducing the length of the background papers, editing them, and preparing the entire manuscript for the compositor. This she performed skillfully and with dispatch.

Finally, we are grateful to the many people in industry who have unstintingly given of their time to listen and react to our ideas, answer our questions, and keep us grounded in reality.

Boston, April 1978   Richard H. Egdahl

Diana Chapman Walsh

Contents

CONTEXT AND ISSUES

Diana Chapman Walsh

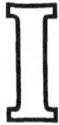

Introduction

1

Three legal developments have set the stage for this volume. Seemingly unrelated and spanning nearly a decade, they have two common attributes: an impact on the availability of information for decisions about health and a strong bearing on the role that private industry will play in health care.

Of the three developments, the newest may have the least immediate impact on industry, but it will be significant as it unfolds over time. The United States Supreme Court, in June 1977, struck down the legal profession's historic ban on advertising[1] and, by implication, perhaps cleared the way for other professionals—including physicians—to advertise their services and even their fees for routine procedures. The New York State Board of Regents, already deeply involved in the issue of professional advertising, quickly followed the Supreme Court's lead and voted in July to allow the physicians and other professionals under the board's jurisdiction to advertise their services through the print media. In September, the Federal Trade Commission opened hearings to investigate charges that organized medicine's policies—particularly those relating to advertising—constitute an unlawful restraint of trade. This chain of events may fundamentally alter the nature of the medical marketplace. How rapidly the change will occur, and whether for the good, is a matter of some controversy. But the inevitability of some change was attested to by one of the New York regents:

> We cannot play King Canute; we cannot hold back the waves. The question is not whether physicians will advertise. The question is how and with what restrictions.
>
>   Emlyn I. Griffith

Industry, as a substantial payer for health care,[2] has more than a passing interest in the answer to Griffith's question, because it raises other broader ones: questions of access to and use of health services and of how much they will cost. These bring industry into the equation and make an everyday issue of one that used to emerge only in a crisis: how does an employee, indeed how does anyone, find a personal physician? Where can the consumer get the information he needs to make a rational choice of a health care provider? Why has information, especially on charges and costs, been elusive, and, perhaps most important, what will happen if and when this is no longer the case?

Moving backward through time, the second of the three legal events came by way of Congress. The 1973 Health Maintenance Organization (HMO) Act,[3] together with subsequent amendments[4] and regulations,[5] includes a "dual choice" provision entitling qualified HMOs to market their plans to companies in their service areas with twenty-five or more employees. As a consequence, an employer approached by a qualified HMO is obligated to offer his employees the option of joining that plan in lieu of taking traditional insurance. In effect, this places the employer in the unaccustomed position of serving as a conduit for information designed to influence employees' choices of health care providers.

The government's purpose in mandating dual choice was to foster HMO growth. Advocates of market-oriented solutions to the problem of health care costs had convinced Congress of the need to develop alternative delivery systems, such as HMOs, that compete for the health care dollar. To survive, alternative delivery systems must succeed rather quickly in getting their message across and recruiting a "critical mass" of members who are relatively healthy or at least not self-selected on the basis of unusually extensive needs for medical care. And the marketers of HMOs realized long ago that their best hope was to break into employee groups through the vehicle of employment-related health insurance. Along with a few notable successes, HMOs have had problems penetrating employee markets. The Carter administration, pressured by health care costs, is actively commending the HMO alternative to the nation's largest employers and is thus pressing the question of the employer's role in assisting employees with their choices of health care providers. This question circles back to the first—how do employees find a personal physician and what should be the employer's role in assisting them? Because the advertising strictures of organized medicine have always been a stumbling block to HMO marketing, removal of this barrier may auger well for the spread of

HMOs, as well as for the employee who needs an access point into, and a roadmap through, the labyrinthian health care delivery system.

The third legal signpost, the oldest and most dramatic of the three, has been slow to have its full impact on health-related communications. Enacted by the 91st Congress, the Occupational Safety and Health Act (OSHAct) of 1970[6] became law in April 1971 and, seven years later, is in some ways only now addressing the massive problem of occupational health hazards. Troubles have beset the administrative bodies created to implement the act—in particular the Occupational Safety and Health Administration (OSHA) and the National Institute of Occupational Safety and Health (NIOSH), together the lead governmental actors in the occupational health drama. But administrative delays aside, the statute did establish the employer's obligation to inform his workers of job-site health hazards. Indeed, many large corporations were struggling with this complex problem long before OSHAct was passed. Now the pressures will continue to build with each new shred of disquieting evidence about hazardous worksite exposure and also as OSHA moves ahead with the development and enforcement of health standards. The worker's right to know will be an intrinsic part of these, according to Eula Bingham, assistant secretary of labor for occupational safety and health:

> OSHA [has been] urged to issue regulations which insure that employees are informed of their exposure to potentially toxic materials. The last two health standards issued by the agency—covering vinyl chloride and coke oven emissions—contain such provisions, as will all future health standards.[7]

The reason, again in Bingham's words, is straightforward:

> Clearly, informing employees of the hazards to which they are exposed is an important element in reducing occupational disease and injury and one of the significant purposes of the Act.[8]

Informing workers about occupational health hazards is an internal responsibility of the firm that is often operationally separate from other concerns about employee health. This is a practical accommodation to the fact that the content and thrust of the occupational health message, and the problems in constructing and disseminating it, are often fundamentally different from those involved in explaining to employees their health insurance coverage or steering them to a provider in the community. The daily demands on managers of employee benefits are largely unrelated to those on the medical department, and the personnel in the two divisions come from entirely different professional streams. On the other hand, some large corporations, such as American Telephone and Telegraph, have convened high-level working groups of managers from the medical, benefits, actuarial, and finance departments to look at the problems of cost and quality in health care, with an eye for solutions that may cut across departmental lines. The traditional separation between occupational and nonoccupational medicine is beginning to blur[9], and many large employers are making an effort, through either the medical or the benefits department, to alert employees to the importance of healthful life-styles and discriminating use of the health care system. It seems logical that the success of these efforts will be contingent to some degree on good employee relations in the industrial health domain. Chapter 6 returns to this issue of the extent to which a corporation's diverse responsibilities and activities related to employees' health can or should be approached as a unitary whole.

Common Threads and Themes

While distinct, the three topics of this volume reinforce one another, because they reflect similar origins and needs in the social and political environment. A need for more information is evident in each of the three areas: if finding a physician can be a challenge for even sophisticated consumers, it is largely for want of appropriate information. When high-quality HMOs are slow to capture an adequate share of the market, the problem can often be traced to difficulty in conveying the positive features of an unfamiliar entity to an uninformed audience. And if assessing and controlling workplace health hazards have strong scientific and technical components, protecting workers from recognized hazards is facilitated greatly by effective education of employees on safe work practices and two-way communication between workers and management on how best to monitor and control the safety of the working environment.

Communication in the three spheres is disrupted by competing forces, some pulling to protect information, others pushing to compel its release. In all three areas, paradoxically, there is at once too much information and too little. We are a society bathed in a sea of information—and misinformation—about health and how to buy it; yet we thirst for a reliable and neutral fact when we are searching for an entry point into the health system.

Conflict in the three areas derives chiefly from the risks—be they tacit or implicit, real or imagined: management's sword of Damocles is the possibility of open-ended legal and financial liability resulting from occupational health hazards; physicians' concerns are that advertising could hurt both the profession and the patient:

> Quite irrespective of what the Federal Trade Commission does or the law decrees, the good and busy docs aren't going to advertise— they have no compulsion to attract more business. And so the rest of these people will be free to advertise. I don't think the profession will be hurt by that, but I think the public might.
>
> Russell B. Roth

The worries Roth alludes to about the integrity and stature of the profession are an undercurrent of much of organized medicine's resistance to advertising. Since a profession's concern over its public image is not a compelling public policy issue, organized medicine usually argues that these issues of professional conduct are fundamental to the trusting physician-patient relationship that is essential for the practice of medicine and must be assiduously protected. But closely related to professional prestige is the issue of income:

Much of the clash that will arise with physician advertising will result from the altered form of competition that will inevitably result in some significant losers, and, of course, they will not be happy.

Lee K. Benham

That some physicians stand to lose seems a nearly inevitable economic consequence of the growing supply of physicians in the United States, discussed at some length in the first volume of this series.[10]

A generalization that emerges from the juxtaposition of the three topics—physician advertising, HMO marketing, and informing workers about occupational hazards—is the extent to which the medical profession has set the boundary conditions—for the consumer's choice of physicians, for the HMO's marketing tactics, and for the occupational physician's domain. Lee Benham has recently argued that organized medicine functions as a "guild" to protect the prerogatives of its members.[8] In all three areas, altruistic concerns about tailoring information to best serve the public interest are conditioned and sometimes overridden by strong economic pressures.

There are real economic risks attendant on releasing information in all three areas and safeguards are clearly needed, along with positive incentives to counterbalance the risks:

> *Both medical practice and occupational health lack the incentives for anyone to generate needed information, and public policies tend to increase the costs to providers who do want to offer information about their practices. It is no simple matter to set up appropriate incentives to information flow, but I would submit that once the legal limitations are overcome—as they now appear to be in the case of physician advertising—then this issue of incentives becomes paramount.*
>
> Lee K. Benham

Measures can be envisaged that would reduce some of the negative incentives and specifically address well-grounded concerns for protection and fair play:

> *One can imagine various protective mechanisms in physician advertising—strong legal sanctions against the misuse of medical information, a kind of Better Business Bureau for medical advertising, or something akin to the National Underwriters' Laboratory. Individual physicians can be assured an opportunity to rebut information that they feel portrays them unfairly. These are some of many ways to start building toward workable safeguards.*
>
> Paul M. Gertman

Gertman's Better Business Bureau could itself become a physicians' guild unless carefully structured to avoid provider domination. Among the most crucial safeguards are those that would protect privacy and confidentiality—inescapable dilemmas in the handling of health information. The individual has a right to privacy until society has an overriding need to know. But at what point the balance tips—when and for what reasons some privacy can be forgone—will hinge strongly on individual assumptions and priorities. Disputes over confidentiality and privacy often derive from basic philosophical conflicts that are not easily resolved. For example, organized labor has recently gone on record supporting the release of employees' health records to the federal government for epidemiological research into workplace health hazards. Management has opposed such disclosures without the employee's written consent, a condition the researchers feel would hopelessly bias their samples. An apparent reversal of traditional roles, this controversy, discussed more fully in chapter 4, seems to find management in the position of defending employees' rights against a government incursion supported by organized labor. The labor viewpoint, however, is that the need to identify workplace health hazards is of paramount concern, and, moreover, that management's access to the information, regardless of how conscientiously it may be handled, has already so completely breached its confidentiality as to render further concern for privacy pointless.

A similarly wide philosophical chasm separates the contending forces in the physician advertising arena, the subject of chapter 2. Physicians who oppose advertising assert their wish to protect patients as well as the broad public interest. Consumer groups argue, to the contrary, that the physician is protecting himself and that his concern for the patient smacks of paternalism and materialism. Distinctions are not always obvious between paternalism on the one hand, with its pejorative connotations, and, on the other, the appropriate exercise of legitimate concern for someone else's well-being, which is, after all, the essence of medicine. Again, drawing those lines is an essentially subjective exercise, based on assumptions about who really controls the information, with what motivation, and to what effect. The tension between paternalism and appropriate concern is a constant undercurrent of the three topics:

> *Even those of us who oppose paternalism and uphold strongly the sovereign rights of the consumer are troubled by this thought: wouldn't it be good if the consumer would make the choice that is in his own best interest? And how can we help him to do that without intruding excessively on his right to choose?*
>
> Sol Levine

Scope of This Volume

Peripheral to the three central topics—physician advertising, HMO marketing, and information about health hazards—are a welter of informational issues in health that must remain beyond the scope of this volume. The breadth of "information" as a concept necessitates a winnowing process, even when it entails arbitrary distinctions. Thus, for example, data management issues emerge only in relation to the three major topics. Little specific attention is given to the collection, aggregation, and use of information that serves, for example, to describe the health status and needs of the employee population, or the health resources available in the corporation and the broader community, or the claims and utilization experience under the employee benefit package. These topics have been touched upon briefly in previous volumes in this series and will be examined more fully in future volumes.

Limited attention is paid the theme of health promotion—the need, now so frequently enunciated, for Americans to reassess their life-styles and the corollary that the worksite offers a natural forum for efforts to put that message across. Unquestionably a communication issue in health, this monumental challenge will for now be left aside, as for the most part will mechanical issues of how to communicate, through what media and channels, with what frequency and what specific message. Technical expertise in this area is well developed in most large firms and can regularly be supplemented through consultants, trade publications, and a steady stream of professional conferences and courses.

The objective of this volume is to raise some new issues and alert industry to still inchoate changes in the environment within which its health programs function. With each successive chapter, management's responsibility becomes progressively more direct, but how best to discharge it remains a dilemma in all three spheres. Also running throughout are these recurrent questions: When information is not readily available, why not? Does the information exist? If so, what risks and benefits might attend its release? What safeguards are needed against misleading or gratuitously damaging information and against invasions of privacy? Where does the responsibility lie for the monitoring of information and the implementation of controls? On what basis can people assess the validity and reliability of information they receive? What are the costs of generating information, who is to bear them and why? At the bottom are basic assumptions about the individual's right to know, the right to self-determination, and most fundamentally of all, about the effects certain kinds of information will have on people, how they will use it, and how it might change them. And all these questions are set against a backdrop of changing societal norms and expectations:

> *People want more and more control over their destinies. They want the information they need to make important judgments, and this is happening on all levels. A lot of forces are fanning these flames—they certainly will not die out.*
>
> Elizabeth M. Kurella

The winds of change are blowing from at least four different directions: social and cultural demands are emanating from the consumerism and self-help movements and are, to some extent, demystifying all the professions. Technological advances—in medicine, in information handling, and in industrial processes—are progressively increasing the stakes of the information game and complicating its rules. Economic pressures are causing a growing feeling that the nation's resources for health care are finite and may be approaching some kind of limit. The political and legal forces, such as the three legal events that have set the stage here, are stimulated principally by the various other pressures and have the effect of repeatedly readjusting and tightening the reins. A few examples of social and cultural pressures serve to establish the broad context; specific technological, economic, and legal developments are elaborated in subsequent chapters.

The Social Context

Whatever other aims may parade at times under the wide banner of "consumerism," both generally and in health, the constant drumbeat is a perceived need for more and better information. In a 1971 symposium volume entitled *The Challenge of Consumerism*, the Conference Board exhorted business to heed the newly raised voice of the consumer in rhetoric that can easily accept words like *physician* and *health care consumer*. For example, in an article by Betty Furness:

> The basic discrepancy between the two sides in the consumer [health] game is information. The [health] consumer can never move intelligently unless he is given the facts. Without being educated, he can't even know how to ask the right questions. Industry [the physician] is not playing fairly unless it [he] makes sure the consumer has all the information he needs.[12]

And later in the same article:

> There is no longer an easy acceptance of corporate [physician] reliability. Consumers are growing more and more suspicious and more and more questioning. The myth that just because a product is on the market [a physician has a license] means it [he] has been tested and proven to be safe [and competent], has been exploded ... People are demanding that the rules ... change. At the top of the list, they want the right to ask questions— and have them answered.[13]

Finally, in a contribution by Mary Gardiner Jones, then a federal trade commissioner:

> What is it basically that [health] consumers want from their marketplace? ... to be taken seriously ... not to be treated as if they have the mentality of twelve ... not to be solely dependent upon the goodwill and honesty of the merchants and manufacturers [physicians and health care providers] with whom they deal ... Today consumers must have completely dispassionate information about all of the transactions to which they are a party.[14]

With similar substitutions, the quotations can also sound like demands on the employer to warn employees of workplace health hazards. The parallels between the rhetoric from the consumer movement of the 1960s and current conflicts over health information link the challenges now facing health providers to those with which industry has been living for some two decades. A brief look at the genesis of the consumer movement is instructive, for just as business was advised in the 1960s to accede to the call for fuller product information, in hopes of harnessing constructively the energy of the consumer movement, so should the health establishment, in and out of industry, meet their new challenges with a more responsive posture.

The consumer movement has many and dispersed roots, going back at least to the civil rights movement of the 1950s. Consumerism came of age during the early 1960s with President Kennedy's consumer protection message to Congress in 1962 and President Johnson's appointment of the first White House adviser on consumer affairs. Events unfolded rapidly thereafter, leading to a kaleidoscopic succession of legislative enactments emphasizing disclosure of information, safety of consumers and workers, and protection of the environment. White House conferences—for example, on food and nutrition, aging, child health—brought consumers to Washington and provided an official forum for their opinions. Federal and state governments, as well as the private sector, have institutionalized the consumer voice in new special-interest entities. Established entities, such as the Federal Trade Commission, have stepped up their consumer protection efforts manyfold.

All these developments reflect changes in the expectations consumers bring to the marketplace, as well as changes in the marketplace itself. Consumers are better educated, more sophisticated, and more critical, but further removed from the sources of production. The marketplace is progressively more complex and varied, with increasing numbers and kinds of options and choices. A component of the consumer's higher expectations is a new emphasis on the quality of life and on the environment.

From these trends has evolved an atmosphere in which OSHAct could pass with only eight dissenting votes, and in which advertising by physicians and marketing by HMOs may seem more appropriate than in the past. The role of consumers in the health care system is a separate but parallel development. Again, with momentum dating back to the 1960s when Office of Economic Opportunity health programs introduced a role for consumers of health services, the consumer movement in health has fanned out into self-help projects, holistic medicine, and into local and regional health planning, where consumers have won an increasingly conspicuous presence.

While consumers have become more involved in health, physicians have had to contend in recent years with persistently bad press. Daniel S. Greenberg dissects the "unflattering picture" painted of the medical profession: "innumerable reports about insurance fraud, needless treatment, dangerous drugs, rapidly rising costs, excess hospital capacity, incompetent physicians who retain their licenses, a potential physician surplus while many areas are underserved, technological extravagances, such as the CAT scanner fad, and so forth."[15] Himself a well-known medical writer, Greenberg muses about the reasons the press has seemed hostile to medicine. His conclusion:

> In recent years, federal interest in health-care policy has spawned, directly and indirectly, a small industry that is concerned with analyzing, and issuing reports on, the economics and administration of health care. . . . All these organizations are problem-seeking groups, devoted to discovering what's wrong and suggesting what might be done about it. . . . And since, in fact, there is a good deal wrong with the distribution, organization and practice of American medicine, they find a good deal to report on.[16]

Problems of access, quality, and cost are real. Chapters 2 and 3 will make the case that they are tightly bound up with issues of information and communication, and will probe possible solutions. Chapter 4 will explore how occupational health hazards create additional communication problems for industry in the context of rapidly increasing knowledge of actual and potential workplace health hazards and a more sophisticated, better educated worker and consumer.

Health Care Advertising and Marketing: The Lady, or the Tiger?

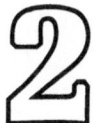

Ethical strictures against advertising are deeply rooted in the history and traditions of the professions. In its June 1977 decision upholding the right of attorneys to advertise, the United States Supreme Court at once acknowledged these historical roots and dismissed them as anachronistic:

> It appears that the ban on advertising originated as a rule of etiquette and not as a rule of ethics . . . But habit and tradition are not in themselves an adequate answer to a constitutional challenge. In this day, we do not belittle the person who earns his living by the strength of his arm or the force of his mind. Since the belief that lawyers are somehow "above" trade has become an anachronism, the historical foundation for the advertising restraint has crumbled.[1]

The courts have given the signal for one of two doors to be opened—one to a more accessible, more responsive, more cost-efficient health system; the other to deceptive advertising, huckstering, and an overmedicalized population. The reader is left to guess which will emerge, the lady, or the tiger? As in the story,[2] no one knows for certain, but all can form an opinion on the available evidence. The short story is a classic because of its exquisite ambiguity. Did the young princess signal the righthand door to consign her splendid lover to a lifetime of happiness with the beautiful competitor she hated, or did she choose instead to send him quickly to his death, where he might "wait for her in the blessed regions of semi-barbaric futurity? . . . The more we reflect on this question, the harder it is to answer."[3] So it may seem with the question of physician advertising and its potential impact on consumers, although the Supreme Court does not share the princess's certain knowledge of the answer, and the alternative outcomes are unlikely to find the health care consumer—the young suitor of our tale—either eaten alive or transported away in bliss. Still our narrative must close, as the short story did, with the question dangling.

We depart from the story's plot, however, to expose our particular bias. We believe that a more informed consumer of health care will question and challenge constructively, and a more competitive marketplace will gain not only efficiency but also variety, sensitivity to consumers' needs, and ultimately more effectiveness—not instantaneously with the opening of a mysterious door, but gradually and incrementally, with concerted efforts on the part of health care providers, payers, and consumers—including private industry—to build safeguards, establish standards, and ensure a positive outcome. But first those deep-seated traditions will need to be examined.

The Past: Advertising and Organized Medicine

Professionals have always thought of themselves as public servants, not as common tradesmen, and have, therefore, disdained commercial conduct, including promotion of their services and solicitation of clients, as unbefitting their station:

> Originally, the professions didn't advertise because they viewed themselves as providing services exclusively. Remuneration was incidental and at the client's discretion, based on his ability to pay and his appraisal of the service rendered. British barristers' robes had a pocket in the back where the client could slip his payment without the barrister's seeing the amount. Unfortunately (or fortunately, depending on your point of view), things have changed, and now professionals usually set fees. The issue has been taken out of the client's hands and I wonder whether that one fundamental change doesn't eliminate any reason for not permitting advertising.
> David B. Hershenson

Enjoinders against solicitation in medicine originated to distinguish the true professional from the huckster and pitchman, who was at the time very much in evidence. Quacks and nostrum makers—or "empirics" as they originally preferred to be called—flourished in eighteenth-century England, spurred on by the newly developed patent system which enabled them to copyright the names of their miracle elixers and salves, and also by a real shortage of physicians which left the public with little choice but to turn either to the local apothecary or to the traveling nostrum promoter for medical advice and assistance.[4]

Milestones in the early history of advertising in England and the United States often consisted of new departures in the promotion of medicinals. In the "first notable example of a mass assault on the public" by advertisers,[5] health was the product being pushed—or rather escape from the ravages of the plague, which peaked in 1665. Daniel Defoe's *Journal of the Plague Year* describes a frightened public, turning to "conjurors and witches" for physic, charms, philtres, exorcisms, incantations, and amulets, and "storing themselves with such Multitudes of Pills, Potions and Preservatives" as to "prepare their bodies for the Plague instead of preserving them against it."[6]

Through most of the eighteenth century, the medicine men sold their myriad "cures" for all sorts of real or imagined conditions through lurid promotional activities in traveling medicine shows and the penny press that was beginning to emerge. Ironically—knowing what we now do—tobaccos and snuffs were among the most aggressively advertised "cure-alls." American medicine was then still deeply in the shadow of England and the nostrums from the mother country were widely and flamboyantly advertised in the fledgling American press throughout the eighteenth and into the nineteenth century. An investment of 10,000 pounds to promote a patent medicine in the late nineteenth century was believed almost certain to return a large fortune.[7]

In 1796 the colonists' own entrepreneurial spirit was unleashed with the creation of the United States Patent Office. The strain of quackery that subsequently developed was even more inventive and ostentatious than its European counterpart. Advertising for patent medicines became the mainstay of the American newspaper industry until the early 1900s when some magazines (led by the *Ladies Home Journal* and *Colliers*) began to campaign against it. After the Pure Food and Drug Act was passed in 1906, the government began to grasp for control over the huckstering medicine men.

Meanwhile, the "true professional" still had a limited armamentarium. Voltaire, the eighteenth-century French philosophe, had characterized a physician as "one who pours drugs of which he knows little into a body of which he knows less."[8] The educational system for ensuring that American physicians at least possessed some practical skills was still grossly inferior to the German or English systems. To improve medical education and advance the quality of care, the American Medical Association was formed; it convened for the first time in Philadelphia in 1847, with the establishment of a code of medical ethics high on the agenda. The code adopted at that meeting evolved into the *Principles of Medical Ethics* which have remained essentially intact through the years, save for occasional revisions to "reflect the temper of the times and the eternal quest to express basic concepts with clarity."[9] It is section 5 of those principles, which says in part, "a physician . . . should not solicit patients,"[10] that is at issue here.

In pursuit of its other mission—the elevation of standards for medical education—the AMA stimulated the promulgation of state licensure requirements for physicians, and, through the famous Flexner Report,[11] submitted to the Carnegie Foundation in 1910, the complete restructuring of the system of medical education. The Flexner Reforms led to the closing of the more than 400 low-quality proprietary medical schools that had sprung up during the early nineteenth century and to the grounding of medical education in a firm academic and scientific base, based principally on the German model. The Flexner Reforms have recently been criticized by some[12,13] for leading American medicine into its high-technology, highly specialized, and some say sterile and dehumanizing mold. But few question that for their time the reforms were needed.

The same can probably be said for the original ethical code. Protecting the public from the quackery that was so rampant was certainly a worthy objective and was a legitimate part of the motivation for roundly condemning solicitation of patients as unprofessional behavior. Many physicians still hold to that principle in a good-conscience belief that it continues to serve the public interest:

> *The profession has always taken the absolute position that there shall be no advertising. Once this is breached, there ensue critical problems of definition and connotation. It was difficult enough to enforce the proscription against all advertising; if it is relaxed I don't know how we are going to enforce standards of truth and fair play to protect the public.*
>
> C. Rollins Hanlon

The most strident critics of organized medicine tend to portray the profession as an outdated guild fighting a last rearguard action to protect its prerogatives and forestall inevitable and salutary change. The stalwarts of organized medicine sometimes inveigh against any governmental intrusion in the affairs of the profession. Somewhere between the extremes is a more balanced perspective that recognizes the nuances and complexities of the arguments on both sides. Changing circumstances have created good reasons for updating the professional rules that have limited the flow of information to the health care consumer, but legitimate grounds remain for concern about the possible consequences.

Updating the Rules for Changing Times

The changing circumstances that have undermined traditional policies on the availability of information about health services have come from various directions, some impinging on medicine from the outside, others percolating up from within.

How Are Times Changing?

Exogenous factors include the social pressures outlined in chapter 1—the consumer movement and related claims on behalf of the individual's "right to know" and a general philosophy calling for freedom of information for its own sake:

The judgment that the consumer makes is sovereign, whether he's purchasing health care or selecting an automobile. It may be true that we don't have all the information we need to make informed purchases of health care, but the same is true for automobiles. The point is that society should be allowed to make its choices without medicine's imposing its view of reality on the rest of us and saying, in effect: "People should not be permitted to choose because we know better than they what is best for them."

R. Hopkins Holmberg

Also coming from the outside are expanded uses of antitrust law and "a growing awareness of the social role of competitive markets . . . as an instrument for achieving 'the best allocation of resources, the lowest prices, the highest quality, and the greatest material progress,' [and] as the central nervous mechanism of a decentralized power structure."[14] These ideas about economic competition are integral to the new emphasis on publicizing information about where to go for health care, and are expanded upon later in this chapter.

Within medicine, increasing specialization—itself the product of a complex of factors and events[15] brought a steady decline in the number of physicians practicing general medicine (from 94 per 100,000 population in 1931 to 56 per 100,000 in 1973).[16] A "hidden system for primary care,"[17] consisting of specialists in internal medicine, pediatrics, and to some extent, obstetrics-gynecology, has largely replaced general practice. Since the system is hidden, finding appropriate entrances can be a real challenge: even sophisticated consumers admit to difficulty finding their way into and successfully negotiating the personal health care system. This is attested to by the president of a state Blue Cross Association:

I'm convinced that we need this public information, because I'm a victim myself, though I've been in the health care business for thirty-one years, and so is the chairman of our board. The physician who took care of my family for years recently died and I've not been able to find a replacement for him. Blue Cross has been under pressure to change the insurance incentives favoring hospital-based care, but quite apart from financial considerations, many people turn to emergency rooms because they don't know where else to go.

Arthur G. Carty

and by the medical director of a major corporation:

When I was in practice I knew all the physicians and their qualifications so I didn't need a directory or fee schedule. But when I later moved to a different community, I found that even the AMA roster of physicians, with its listings of credentials, didn't tell me how particular physicians handled patients or what I really needed to know. Bill Cosby likes to say that he has visions of developing appendicitis and choosing a surgeon who turns out to have been a whiz on gall bladders but to have flunked appendectomies. In essence, that's the problem we all face.

Bruce W. Karrh

The two comments raise ancillary issues that are treated more fully below—the financing of health services and how that affects patterns of use; and the fundamental dilemma of defining quality of care and how it relates to credentials.

Another of the internal factors that is pressing medicine to disseminate more information about where consumers may go for care is the growing role of high technology. The "technological imperative,"[18] combined with extensive third-party coverage for care and rising consumer expectations, feeds "a tendency to take action, whatever the cost, if it offers even a slight possibility of utility."[19] Costs rise as a result, and "the ethic of doing everything possible [becomes] increasingly unrealistic in the face of biomedical advances."[20] At this point, medical sociologist David Mechanic argues, some sort of rationing becomes necessary, either overtly, by administrative fiat, or implicitly, by limiting resources and thus forcing providers to make difficult allocation decisions. The need for trade-offs and triage confounds the traditional medical rule that the physician does everything possible for each of his patients with no thought to societal consequences. This makes it all the more important that consumers be informed about the availability and limitations of various medical procedures, so that they can participate in the decisions that must be made.

The most immediate impetus to changing information policies in health is the dilemma of rising costs, treated in some detail in the first volume of this series. The cost problem is a corollary of the technological imperative and of the issue of access to care, both of which have major informational dimensions:

> One of the principal products of the health system is information and one of the worst inequities is in the amount of information different people have.
>
> Lee K. Benham

During the 1960s, the decade in which Medicare and Medicaid were enacted, access to personal health services was the preeminent public policy objective. Policies addressing access to care derive chiefly from concern about social inequality; the financing and service programs of the 1960s attempted to redistribute resources for health care, ensure the availability of acceptable services without financial barriers, and redress some of the gross inequities that were known to exist. Those efforts have brought substantial improvement, although access is still a real problem for millions of Americans who fall through one or another of the cracks between private and public financing programs. But the efforts to improve access have temporarily been eclipsed by the complex cost problems they helped to create.

Cost containment approaches have taken many forms, some—like certificate of need, manpower policies, and health planning—addressing the supply side of the equation, some—like cost sharing, utilization review, and health promotion—the demand side. Each of these regulatory interventions seeks control over a specific element of the system. Justifying the interventions is the observation that the market for health services is flawed—because providers control demand, third-party payment insulates consumers and providers from the economic consequences of purchasing decisions, and consumers are ignorant of the prices charged for various services and of possible alternatives.

In opposition is the view that consumer ignorance is either exaggerated[21] or is largely an artifact:

> *A lot of consumer ignorance is artificial in that the profession and state governments have repressed the availability of information, on the assumption, I suppose, that a little knowledge is a dangerous thing. Of course the consumer is abysmally ignorant in many ways, but not only in health care matters. To have a market system that works tolerably well, it isn't necessary to have every consumer perfectly informed in every choice he makes. The real value of a functioning market, with information freely available, is that it sets up incentives that operate across the board on all providers and benefit all consumers, even the most ignorant. Markets cater primarily to the marginal consumer, who is apt to be better informed.*
> Clark C. Havighurst

From this it would seem to follow that to solve the problem of health care costs, government should try to limit its interventions to those that will shore up the private market and encourage competition. And, as Havighurst implies, one of the crucial steps toward a working market is to break the logjam of consumer information about where to purchase services.

Not everyone agrees. The quotations in the box show the range of opinion evoked by the notion that information has been suppressed. In addition, market forces are not universally subscribed to as the answer. For example, Anne and Herman Somers are "doubtful that the notion that there can be effective price competition among doctors in the medical marketplace will stand up." and believe that efforts to promote competition might more fruitfully be focused on the nonpayroll items purchased by hospitals (drugs, appliances, equipment, consultative and housekeeping services) and on consumer purchases of prescription drugs and applicances.[22] A recent report by the Congressional Budget Office also expresses skepticism because a "lack of knowledge and limited advertising are not new phenomena and therefore do not explain the recent more rapid growth in health care costs."[23] The report goes on to suggest that attempts to establish price as an influence on health services should seek not only to improve consumer knowledge but should also change the insurance and tax systems which make consumption decisions insensitive to price.

Advocates of market-oriented solutions are led by the supporters of various alternative delivery systems, such as HMOs, and some others as well. One example is Stanford University Professor Alain C. Enthoven. In a proposed national health insurance scheme, submitted at the request of Health, Education, and Welfare Secretary Joseph Califano, Enthoven argues for assuring that all people have choices among competitive alternatives and that they have good information on which to base their choices.[24] Another example comes from an unexpected source. The American Medical Association's National Commission on the Cost of Medical Care recently issued a forward-looking report which acknowledged the need for substantial regulation of health services, recognized weaknesses in both public utility and market-strengthening regulations, and concluded that the answer "lies in strengthening price consciousness in the health care marketplace ... [and providing] a greatly enhanced decision-making role for the consumer."[25] The entire report seems at

CONSUMER IGNORANCE? PROVIDER SUPPRESSION? . . . OR SOMETHING MORE PERPLEXING?

Rick J. Carlson: The argument seems to be that the consumer shouldn't know because he would fail either to understand or to use the information appropriately. The irony is that in withholding information, physicians are handicapping themselves. If consumers had more information about health, the medical care system and physicians individually would benefit profoundly, I suspect, because one of physicians' major problems these days comes from the unreasonable expectations Americans bring to the medical encounter. It's perplexing, therefore, to see the medical profession taking the position that people shouldn't have information.

C. Rollins Hanlon: We are talking about two constituencies—physicians and patients—and they have a relationship. I don't believe the adversary relationship Mr. Nader advocates is a way to straighten out a problem. I'd like to think of it as a partnership, even for selfish, economic reasons.

Michael D. Bromberg: It's not a partnership, though, if one partner has the choice of withholding information from the other. The question is how do we get enough information to the consumer so that he can be a real partner?

Dr. Hanlon: I take strong exception to this notion that physicians have been guilty of repression or conspiracy. Perhaps more information is needed—the ultimate being that physicians would conduct mini medical schools in their offices and try to make every patient as much an expert in his particular illness as the physician himself. It is the one billion person-to-person contacts that take place in physicians' offices around this country every year that matter, not directories, posters, or commercials. Those of us who spend many hours explaining things to patients are willing to admit that we sometimes still fail in this task. So I might grant inadequacy of information, perhaps. But conspiracy? Utter nonsense!

John N. Tulley: As an involved layman, I often hear it said that the medical profession's clear choice not to air its dirty laundry in public suggests that something is perhaps being hidden—that other members of the club or guild are being protected. The layman's perception is that a physician is much more likely to be thrown out of the medical society for posing an economic threat to some other physician's practice than for performing too many unnecessary operations—however that is defined. If the profession wants its peer review mechanism accepted, some educated "consumers" must be permitted in behind those closed doors. Because right now people don't know what's going on there and so they are drawing inferences and the inferences, overall, are not favorable to the profession.

Willis B. Goldbeck: That's a terribly important point. Much of the pressure to loosen the physician's grip on advertising is coming from the public's perception of a profession withholding information. I say that with no particular concern as to how true that impression may be. The perception is the significant fact.

Alasdair C. MacIntyre: I think the problem about medicine in America is not a problem about physicians. It's a problem about the American public—about the definition of medical need by the public. And "the public," of course, is an amorphous term. To illustrate, recently I turned on my television for a short stretch of time and saw in succession, advertisements from the American Heart Association, the American Diabetes Association, and the American Cancer Association. There is something insane about this. For every one of these causes in isolation a very good case can be made, but the notion that I ought to be worrying all the time about whether to give my money to cure cancer or stop heart disease or so on—something has gone very badly wrong. These advertisements cost a lot of money. They are there only because they are productive and they point to this insatiable American public demand for medical care. I don't see any possibility of the medical profession's reforming the whole situation; it will have to be a much larger change.

odds with official AMA policy, and nowhere more so than on the issue of information for consumers. The AMA is locked in battle with the Federal Trade Commission over this issue and the chairman of the AMA board of trustees portrays the struggle in Armageddon terms:

> The Federal Trade Commission says they will create our code of ethics for us and they will determine whether or not we are abiding by it ... The whole nature of medicine hangs on this issue and we are resolved to fight it just as long and just as hard as we possibly can and not settle for anything less than prevailing in our own viewpoint.[26]

The AMA-FTC stand-off has emerged out of a series of legal redefinitions of public policy on professional advertising.

Changing the Rules

In the past two years the United States Supreme Court has handed down three decisions that have eroded the foundations of organized medicine's ethical constraints on advertising and solicitation and heightened its vulnerability to the FTC's rising tide of interest in the medical marketplace.

First, in *Goldfarb v. Virginia State Bar*[27] the court found in 1973 that a state bar's minimum fee schedule for a particular legal transaction violated federal antitrust law. The decision was important because it denied the "learned professions" an exemption they had hitherto seemed to enjoy from antitrust liability.

In 1976, the court heard *Virginia Board of Pharmacy v. Virginia Citizens Consumer Council*[28] and ruled that a pharmacist's right to advertise prescription drug prices was protected by the first amendment. Emphasizing the value of advertising to individuals for important life decisions and to society in a free market economy, the ruling extended the constitutional protection of free speech to "commercial speech," that is, advertising, and cleared the way for the *Bates* decision on advertising by attorneys.

In *Bates et al v. State Bar of Arizona*,[29] decided June 27, 1977, the court ruled in a close (5–4) decision that a state's prohibition of advertising by attorneys was unconstitutional. The case involved newspaper advertising of fees for routine legal services. How much further the ruling extends—within the legal profession and beyond—is open to legal interpretation. The court reserved judgment here, stating that particular issues raised in different professions and the general question of electronic media advertising might have to be considered individually. Stiff and Bloom, in part II of this volume, hazard some predictions on these unresolved issues and point out that the legality of quality claims and in-person solicitation are also still in doubt. How "routine services" will be defined and what limits can be placed on advertising for nonroutine procedures remain ambiguous. This clouds the issue of the conditions under which physicians will be permitted to advertise their fees:

> I don't think the Supreme Court is going to allow a great deal of fee advertising by physicians. Few services will be classified as "rou-

tine," I expect, and therefore appropriate for fee advertising. The dissenting opinions in Bates expressed great concern that fee advertising may be inherently deceptive and I suspect that future decisions—particularly on physician advertising—will see this concern prevail.

Paul N. Bloom

I read the decision and I just cannot agree. I had a chance to discuss this decision with Justice Blackmun recently and my very strong impression was that lawyers are now perfectly free to advertise except through television and radio.

George R. Dunlop

Clarification of these ambiguities will move along three major avenues. First, the courts will doubtless continue to play a major role in the controversy. Second, some state licensure authorities have already begun to revise their regulations to reflect the Bates decision. The New York State Regents led the way because the United States Supreme Court's decision in June was announced while they were independently nearing completion of a total recodification of their rules defining professional conduct. The Regents have jurisdiction over thirty learned professions in New York—all except law and theology. Despite the specificity of Bates to the legal profession, the Regents had little doubt of its relevance to other professions and quickly integrated its principles into the new rules—in a unanimous decision announced just one month later. Griffith and Abbott, in part II, describe the Regents' deliberations and the position they finally adopted.

The third path to clarification will be through the ethical codes of the various professional societies. In medicine, of course, the national body is the AMA, which recently liberalized its official stance on advertising. The liberalization was passed in April 1976, well before the Bates decision, but after the AMA was charged by the FTC, in December 1975, with violating the Sherman Antitrust Act by, among other alleged activities, suppressing the flow of information. Excerpts from the 1976 reinterpretation, together with the 1972 version it superseded, appear in the box. The Supreme Court cited the 1976 AMA guidelines in support of the Bates ruling. But some—including the FTC—argue that the liberalization is just window dressing: a public pronouncement by the beleagured national organization, with little impact anticipated on local level reality. This is one of the issues the FTC investigation will seek to resolve.

Organized medicine does give substantial autonomy to state and county societies for revision and enforcement of ethical canons. A philosophical shift at the national level remains largely symbolic until it works its way into the thinking of the local leadership, where control of sanctioning mechanisms resides. The ultimate sanction the society can exercise is to expel the offending member, but the FTC contends that this action can theoretically set in motion a domino effect with potentially serious economic sequelae, such as loss of hospital privileges and of referrals, denial of specialty certification or state reciprocity, loss of malpractice coverage or greatly increased premiums.

ADVERTISING AND THE ETHICAL PHYSICIAN —THE AMA CODE

From the Principles of Medical Ethics, 1957, Section 5:

"A physician may choose whom he will serve . . . He should not solicit patients."

Solicitation of Patients, Direct or Indirect
"Solicitation of patients, directly or indirectly, by a physician, or by groups of physicians, is unethical. This principle protects the public from the advertiser and salesman of medical care by establishing an easily discernible and generally recognized distinction between him and the ethical physician. Among unethical practices are included the not always obvious devices of furnishing or inspiring newspaper or magazine comments concerning cases in which the physician or group or institution has been, or is, concerned. Self-laudations defy the traditions and lower the moral standard of the medical profession; they are an infraction of good taste and are disapproved." . . .

Acceptable Advertising
"The most worthy and effective advertisement possible, even for a young physician, especially among his brother physicians, is the establishment of a well-merited reputation for professional ability and fidelity. This cannot be forced, but must be the outcome of character and conduct." . . .

Solicitation of Patients by Groups
"The Council is unable to see any difference in principle between a group of physicians advertising themselves under whatsoever title they may assume and an individual physician advertising himself."

Extreme penalties are rare, however, and one of the questions that the advertising issue raises is how effectively the profession has policed its members.

After the litigious dust has settled, the professional societies will doubtless revise their codes and procedures, for example, as Stiff and Bloom suggest in part II, to include a "glossary of acceptable terms" that members can use in advertising. The dust is still being stirred, however, by the FTC in its several investigations of the health professions. The outcome of these cases, which may find their way to the Supreme Court, will eventually establish the ground

From the Statement of the Judicial Council, April 9, 1976

"*Advertising*—The Principles do not proscribe advertising: they proscribe the solicitation of patients. Advertising means the action of making information or intention known to the public. The public is entitled to know the names of physicians, the type of their practices, the location of their offices, their office hours, and other useful information that will enable people to make a more informed choice of physician.

"The physician may furnish this information through the accepted local media of advertising or communication, which are open to all physicians on like conditions. Office signs, professional cards, dignified announcements, telephone directory listings, and reputable directories are examples of acceptable media for making information available to the public.

"A physician may give biographical and other relevant data for listing in a reputable directory ... If the physician, at his option, chooses to supply fee information the published data may include his charge for a standard office visit or his fee or range of fees for specific types of services, provided disclosure is made of the variable and other pertinent factors affecting the amount of the fee specified. The published data may include other relevant facts about the physician, but false, misleading or deceptive statements or claims should be avoided.

"*Solicitation*—The term "solicitation" in the Principles means the attempt to obtain patients by persuasion or influence, using statements or claims that (1) contain testimonials, (2) are intended or likely to create inflated or unjustified expectations of favorable results, (3) are self-laudatory and imply that the physician has skills superior to other physicians engaged in his field or specialty of practice, or (4) contain incorrect or incomplete facts, or representations or implications that are likely to cause the average person to misunderstand or be deceived ..." Editors' note: These are excerpts. The full text is available from the Office of the General Counsel, American Medical Association, 535 North Dearborn Street, Chicago, Illinois 60610.

rules for how closely professional organizations will be allowed to circumscribe the activities of their members for the purpose of "upholding ethical standards." The FTC was created sixty-two years ago to protect the public from unfair and deceptive practices. In the past much maligned for moving slowly and without much effect, the commission has been strengthened in recent years by a supportive Congress; appropriations have increased about 15 percent annually over the past ten years.[30]

Since the 1975 *Goldfarb* case did away with the learned profession's exemption, the FTC has cast a wide net into health care delivery and financing practices, fishing for antitrust violations in the prescription drug and eyeglass industries, in the Blue Shield program, and in various activities of the dental and medical professions. The FTC has alleged that the professions' accreditation and certification controls over medical and dental education have restricted entry into and competition within these professions. In 1976 two specialty societies, the American College of Obstetricians and Gynecologists and the American Academy of Orthopedic Surgeons, and, in 1977 a third, the American College of Radiology, signed consent decrees with the FTC, agreeing to discontinue use of "relative value scales" which list comparative numerical values for surgical or medical procedures. Values can be translated to a fee schedule by means of a dollar conversion factor—in the FTC's view making them tantamount to price fixing. The societies disagreed but acceded to the consent order to avoid expensive litigation.

One of the dilemmas that will surface with regard to relative values is that certain types of HMO—particularly the individual practice association (IPA), where participating physicians practice in their offices on a modified fee-for-service basis[31]—must use a fee schedule or the equivalent to establish premiums that are actuarily sound. Since the FTC is in the business of promoting competitive markets and HMOs are viewed as one of the major instruments for infusing some competition into the health care market, it is unclear how the FTC will resolve the conflict that could develop if a very successful IPA were to win a large share of a market.

The advertising complaints against the AMA and the American Dental Association (ADA) follow in the same vein as two of the FTC's earliest probes in health, which challenged prohibitions of advertising price and other information for eyeglasses and prescription drugs. Reinecke, in part II, supplemented by Benham's earlier research,[32] sketches the major issues in the eyeglass industry, but Stiff and Bloom assert that tangible goods like eyeglasses and drugs raise vastly different advertising problems than do intangible medical services, which may be inherently less susceptible to market forces.

Nevertheless, the FTC argued in hearings that began September 7, 1977, that restraints on advertising have inhibited innovation in health care delivery and elevated health care costs. The defendants in the case are the AMA, the Connecticut State Medical Society, and the New Haven County Medical Society, the latter selected to represent the AMA's fifty state societies and 2,000 or so local organizations.

In its defense, the AMA argues in part that the FTC's charge is invalidated by the 1975 liberalization of the advertising rules, permitting all but deceptive advertising. "If being against false and misleading advertising violates the Federal Trade Commission laws," AMA counsel Newton Minnow (the former federal communications commissioner who characterized television as a "vast wasteland") is quoted as having said to the hearing judge, "then I would submit to you that probably the Ten Commandments violate the Federal Trade Commission."[33]

The hearings concluded in March 1978 with an initial decision by administrative law Judge Ernest Barnes anticipated sometime between September and December 1978. If Barnes rules in the FTC's favor, the AMA plans to appeal; whatever the immediate outcome, the controversy over what constitutes misleading advertising is far from settled. Direct relevance to industry is suggested by the fact that one of the alleged anticompetitive actions involves industrial health; the FTC cited the case of an industrial physician in Connecticut who was censured by the medical society for calling on large corporations to become interested in establishing health care programs for their employees. Indirectly, the case is important for industry because of the broad implications it could conceivably have for the costs and quality of personal health services and how they are delivered.

The Present: Practices, Problems, and Progress

The possible impact of relaxed advertising rules on health professionals needs to be seen in the context of the information now available to consumers selecting a provider, whether a primary care physician or dentist, a specialist, a hospital, or some other institution.

Searching for and Selecting Primary Physicians and Dentists

Evidence suggests that people seldom change personal physicians and normally find themselves in the position of choosing one only when their circumstances change or their physician becomes unavailable. But these situations are increasingly common in today's mobile society. Sociologists have shown that lay-referral systems—relatives, neighbors, co-workers, and other friends—are often important in decisions of this nature[34], but our concern here is the *public* information available for the decision. The amount of such information has increased exponentially in the past decade or so and a whole literature has grown up on how to find, select, evaluate, and relate to a personal physician. Two of many possible illustrations are Keith W. Sehnert's 1975 book, *How to Be Your Own Doctor (Sometimes)*[35] and Marvin S. Belsky's *How to Choose and Use Your Doctor.*[36] Both are written by physicians and include a checklist of factors to consider, some objective (education, specialty, board certification, hospital and university affiliations, type of practice, etc.), some subjective (personality, ambiance of office, etc.). Popular magazines commonly run articles in this genre. A book called *Take Care of Yourself*[37] is being purchased in bulk by some carriers and employers and distributed at cost or free to employees. Armco Steel, for example, has disseminated about 10,000 copies.

In addition, the Yellow Pages have grown more useful because specialty listings have become widely accepted and were ruled ethical in a 1975 AMA policy statement. Telephone listing by medical specialty began in Milwaukee about ten years ago but started spreading widely only in about 1974. Now it is done in more than half of the nineteen affiliates of the Bell System.[38] Some controversy has arisen over the specialty headings to be used (whether, for example, weight control, holistic medicine, and other marginal specialties should be included) and some physicians argue that the listings inappropriately encourage patients to diagnose their own problems and self-refer to specialists. Telephone company surveys indicate that in a year some 35 million adults average nearly eight uses each of the "Physicians and Surgeons" listing in the Yellow Pages.[39] But the specialty listings provide only one of several bits of information a potential patient should have.

The next step is a directory, often compiled by the profession and providing somewhat more information by which to compare physicians. For example, the Professional Guild of Arizona published *The Doctors Directory*[40] which defines the twenty-two specialties it lists, groups physicians by specialty and geographic area (with maps) and includes: medical school, specialty training and certifications, with dates; hospital affiliations; office hours; languages spoken; address, telephone number, and public transportation routes; and charges for initial office visit, follow-up visits, and the use of certain procedures and services.

More informative still are the directories published by consumer groups. The *Directory of Evanston Primary Care Physicians*,[41] compiled by the Consumer's Health Group of Evanston, Illinois, provides all the information appearing in the Arizona directory, and: the physician's special interests; research and teaching activities; support personnel; availability of after-office hours; time required to get first and subsequent appointments; office equipment and charge; whether the physician regularly prescribes drugs by generic name and advises patients of possible side effects of drugs. A separate section on "fees and billing" states what the charge is for a routine office visit, whether the physician charges to fill out medical insurance forms, whether he or she accepts Medicaid and Medicare patients, how soon after the visit the bill is due and whether and when unpaid bills are referred to a collection agency. Under the heading "specialty practice information" are listed facts like "phone calls from patients accepted during office hours; anytime for an emergency," or "supportive of women who choose natural childbirth and breast feeding," or "neither performs nor refers patients for abortions . . . does not prescribe intrauterine devices." The directory includes a profile of each of the hospitals in the area and advises readers, "when choosing a primary care physician, you are also choosing a hospital . . . You may want to consider this . . . when selecting a physician." A short glossary is also included, along with an "experience form" on which readers are requested to report on "the usefulness of the Directory . . . [and] your reaction to any given physician."[42]

On the whole, even the most probing directories represent conservative, temperate approaches to disseminating information about physicians' services. Directories have uses and limitations. On the credit side, they bring together rudimentary information on fees and services not conveniently available elsewhere and do so in a format lending itself to comparisons among providers. They save consumers the time and money it would cost to search out the information independently, were they so inclined and had they the skills and resources. With the concrete information they provide, the directories also tend to communicate a philosophy about the virtues of becoming critical "activated patients"[43] and the appropriateness of asking about fees. By training a spotlight on routine fees, the directories—and other forms of fee advertising—might conceivably bring grossly aberrant fees into line and might place a symbolic "ceiling" on rapid cost increases:

> *Lowering of costs seems unlikely, but might not widespread advertising restrain increases by keeping physicians in line and making them reluctant to raise their fees considerably above publicly regarded standard prices?*
>
> Paul M. Gertman

There is disagreement on this point, however; some say experience has shown that ceilings become floors:

> *History has shown what happens when fees are standardized. Almost instantaneously after the schedules are published, the ceiling fee becomes the floor. The lesson is clear—if stabilization of prices is a good idea, you still have to stop and consider whether you are stabilizing them at higher or lower levels.*
>
> Russell B. Roth

> *I have a different perspective on standard fee schedules. As an actuary I work with plans that publish fee schedules of participating providers—that's not an unusual concept. There are some misconceptions here. A published "usual and customary" will in fact become a floor, not a ceiling, because no one will charge less. Moreover, if you peg your fee schedule to be highly competitive—perhaps 10 percent below prevailing—you may draw providers to somewhat lower fees.*
>
> Harold Gilbert

Sometimes it is argued that directories are difficult or costly to keep up to date:

> *The Regional Medical Program experience demonstrated that directories are immensely expensive to collate and to keep up to date, and they are still susceptible to inaccuracy because physicians retire and move and economic forces dictate changes in prices.*
>
> Russell B. Roth

However, Paul Gertman asserts that modern information technology can easily obviate these problems:

> *Information technology is rapidly changing. Within the decade we are clearly going to have statewide data bases with central computers storing physician experience, publications, and a lot of other data. It's not farfetched to predict that, if some of the legal barriers were removed, PSRO-type data could be available over computer lines to corporations, local plants, and even individuals at home. By punching in over a telephone line from a personal*

home computer the individual could access data on the kinds of procedures individual physicians had done and the complication rates, all current and valid within about three months.

As currently conceived, directories still fall far short of answering all the questions a potential consumer of health care ought to be able to ask. They still leave Bruce Karrh to wonder how a given physician relates to his patients and do not assure Bill Cosby that his surgeon is accomplished in "appendectomy."

How much more can we expect of open advertising? It is too soon to predict with confidence. Few physicians and other health professionals are advertising and those leading the way seem to come from the other end of the spectrum from the well-modulated and informative tenor of the directories. Two chiropractors in Florida have already begun advertising on television, a medium some observers worry may be wholly inappropriate for promotion of an individual practitioner's services. The chiropractors are being prosecuted by their state board, and the American Civil Liberties Union is defending them in court.[44] A Virginia surgeon, H. Barry Jacobs, has mailed out thousands of brochures with the come-on "are you tired of paying for your doctor's Cadillac and country club?" and suggesting that his services are more moderately priced. Meanwhile, the most lurid current examples of physician advertising come from California, where, Rick Carlson says, "a lot of crazy things begin, and a few of them stick."

A few Los Angeles entrepreneurs in plastic surgery have taken out display newspaper advertisements promising instant beauty and a happier life, as certified by "before and after" photographs of satisfied customers sporting thicker hair, straighter noses, flatter abdomens, or larger breasts, "You don't have to be rich . . . to make the most of yourself," one of the ads reads over the picture of a reclining bikini-clad model. "Cosmetic surgery can give you what nature didn't . . . breast, face, eyelids, nose, ears, chin, neck, thighs, tummy, etc. Private insurance accepted. Credit arranged. Look your best. You owe it to yourself."[45] In some cases now coming to light, patients have not only been subtly misled but have been maimed and abused.[46] The tone of these campaigns harks back to the early promises for patent medicines; the tragic effects seem to support the most serious misgivings about possible consequences of unrestrained physician advertising:

> *There's definitely danger in physician advertising—not because it's physicians but because it's advertising and we know what advertising does in shaping human behavior. We have to face up to the fact that advertising induces an awful lot of purchases of an awful lot of things that aren't good for anyone. Advertising—even effective advertising—may not provide any valuable information. The one good thing even bad advertising may do is give the consumer a basis for complaining or challenging or questioning. There are legal controls on advertising. These may prove to be an effective weapon in the consumer quiver.*
>
> Willis B. Goldbeck

Goldbeck's suggestion that advertising could serve to protect unwary consumers by providing objective evidence that the promise fell short of the product seems to hold up in the California case. The advertisements in question are deplorable because they trade on insecurity and unhappiness, create false expectations, and sometimes deliver bitter disappointment. Hoping to offer the FTC a disquieting glimpse into the Pandora's box it would open, the AMA presented testimony in the FTC's advertising hearings by a few of these plastic surgeons' victims. Compelling though the testimony is, it may be a two-edged sword for organized medicine's cause, successfully demonstrating that unrestrained advertising can be harmful but also casting doubt on the efficacy of the profession's existing internal controls. Where, one wonders, is the professional self-policing that should have prevented these California tragedies or at least moved with dispatch to forestall their recurrence? Again, the basic issue is quality control—the question that flows from Goldbeck's observation is whether higher quality information about health care services might begin to smoke out differences in quality of care and lead ultimately to overall improvements. Until such information is more widely available, this will remain an open question.

Organized dentistry has more relentlessly than medicine held to the paradigm of the independent, solo, fee-for-service practitioner. Boffa and Rabner, in part II, describe the relative lack of enthusiasm with which the profession has greeted prepaid dentistry. The ADA has been charged by the FTC with anticompetitive behavior paralleling that alleged of the AMA, and when the Supreme Court handed down its decision in *Bates,* the ADA instructed its member societies to desist from prosecuting members who advertised.[47]

Dentistry has its own history of flamboyant advertising, epitomized perhaps by "Painless Parker" who ballyhooed his virtues on billboards and handbills all over California. Now some of his more subdued later twentieth-century bretheren are again turning to advertising and, according to accounts in the *New York Times*[48] and the *Washington Post,*[49] are finding that it pays. A Long Island dentist, for example, reported that advertising had caused his practice volume to jump by "500 percent."[50]

In medicine there are real grounds for concern that advertising will rapidly stimulate inappropriate demand and excessive use of medical services by feeding the "overmedicalization" already rampant in American society. This danger may be somewhat more remote in the case of dentistry, at least until third-party payment becomes more widespread than it now is. There are good arguments for covering some dentistry in a benefit package, for example, the assertion by the director of dental marketing for Blue Cross that 100 million lost work hours can be traced to dental diseases.[51] But because untreated dental disease is quite prevalent in the population, the introduction of dental insurance is costly at first:

> My client company wrote a major new contract for dental services
> in New York City a few years ago. Utilization went up 30 percent
> each of the next two years. The cost per procedure stayed constant
> and people clearly got a lot more dental care. I don't know if they
> got better care or had better dental health at the end, but the
> practitioners in the plan went to union meetings, drummed up

business, and clearly demonstrated that if you remove financial barriers and open up the market there will be an expansion of services.

Harold Gilbert

The FTC's case against the ADA has been scheduled to follow the AMA hearings. The outcome for dentistry will probably depend in part on how the physician case is resolved.

Secondary Providers and Third-Party Payers

Hospitals are beginning to strike out on a different tack—in search of consistently high occupancy rates and more secure budgets. In the past physicians' control over the important purchasing decisions in health simplified the marketing task, which could be targeted almost exclusively to physicians. The pharmaceutical industry developed a system of face-to-face salesmanship to physicians augmented by extensive advertising in medical and professional journals. Medical specialists seeking to build up a practice knew to join the organizations and make the contacts necessary to break into their colleagues' referral networks. Hospitals, until very recently, observed the same rules. They engaged in low-key competition for physicians—the source of admissions— simply by functioning as "the doctor's workshop" complete with the newest equipment and gadgets and a wide enough range of services to provide a congenial and productive professional milieu to attract and hold the kinds of physicians desired for the staff. Meanwhile, the public relations department sent subdued messages into the community, chiefly to raise funds which enabled the hospital to continue making the improvements necessary to satisfy the medical staff and their patients and the hospital trustees as well. All these objectives remain, but with an important new added dimension. Now in many locations there are excess hospital beds, so that oblique competition for physicians is no longer the road to survival. Hospitals have begun to compete directly for patients and indirectly for the "respectable" occupancy rates— often 85 to 90 percent or more—that tend to be a requisite when it comes time to petition for the franchise that certificate-of-need programs are authorized to award or deny, or to plead for rate increases to a rate-setting commission.

More information, be it price, utilization, or similar data is becoming available and the real drive will be through various public media to interpret the objective information. We are seeing the first wave of that now, and the hospital industry is leading the way because that is where there is now a competitive crunch. The ground rules we set for the hospital sector will, I believe, set some precedents for individual providers.

Paul M. Gertman

Two basic kinds of hospital advertising are emerging: one directly selling services and recruiting "customers," the other raising issues and making the hospital's case before the public. In the first instance, a growing number of institutions are using the print media, direct mail, radio, even television, to promote particular services among potential patients. Investor-owned Sunrise Hospital in Las Vegas is among the more visible. Its heavily advertised "recuperative Mediterranean cruise for two" offers patients signing into the hospital on a Friday or Saturday a chance to enter a weekly drawing for the vaunted cruise. The objective is to increase the hospital's weekend patient census; backing the campaign costs the hospital $10,000 a month but, the advertisement asserts, "by encouraging patients to choose to be admitted on the weekend we can better balance our workload, make greater use of available facilities and, in turn, keep our costs down."[52] Other hospitals have had full color supplements inserted in Sunday newspapers, mailed thousands of flyers or booklets into the surrounding community describing how the hospital "serves" it, or advertised particular programs, such as alcohol treatment units. Recognizing the trend, the American Hospital Association has written new guidelines for hospital advertising.

The issue of hospitals' overtly marketing their services has evolved over the past three to four years from one of whether and why to one of how: trade magazines are now full of marketing advice, special courses are being offered, and experts are being brought on to hospital staffs to guide them into "a marketing future." Giller, in part II, discusses some possible implications for the health care industry and for patients. Goldbeck foresees in the trend some potentially helpful implications for large employers:

> Employers and labor unions in many communities do represent a fairly substantial chunk of a hospital's revenues, particularly if they aggregate, and I wonder why hospitals couldn't market to employers and through them to employees on the basis of cost control efforts—"We don't take Friday admissions for Monday surgery," or "We provide peer review for all types of services and all classes of patients." Are we willing to take it a step further and envision the next AEtna ad singling out a hospital that is doing a particularly effective job containing costs, and by implication clearly attempting to influence people to use that hospital instead of another one?
>
> Willis B. Goldbeck

> I'm a very strong advocate of advertising by hospitals for one big reason: doctors make the decisions and I believe that the safest, fairest, and best way to change the health system is through consumer pressure on the physician. The consumer is the only person who can change the way a doctor practices medicine. For example, a lot of physicians have privileges in several hospitals. Suppose one of the hospitals went to one of these corporate consumers and said "Look, there are four hospitals in town. We'll put our quality up against anyone—you decide on that. But we're going to offer you a 5 percent discount. Maybe we're not ready for an HMO yet or maybe we're competing against an HMO. And the corporation looks into it and decides the quality is good, the outcomes are O.K. What's wrong with a 5 percent discount? So the hospital advertises the discount for company employees. I think that's healthy because

> the patient will say to the physician: "Wait a minute. If you put me
> in the hospital whose ad I saw I'll get a 5 percent rebate or my
> company will. Can't you put me there?" That approach makes
> sense to me not only to help educate the patient in making his
> decision but also to get the patient involved in encouraging the
> doctor to become more cost conscious and to change a little bit—
> not by laws and regulations and mandates but by listening to his
> patient—he does that all the time.
>
> Michael D. Bromberg

The AEtna advertisements to which Goldbeck refers epitomize the
"issues advertising" that is now flourishing in the health care field. Again this
is not entirely new; advertisements to justify a particular stand in a health
controversy were an integral part of the malpractice crisis when it peaked in
1975 with the California and New York physician strikes,[53] and have for many
years been used by organized medicine to counter the threat of "socialization."
According to a recent newsletter account, the AMA has announced plans to
wage a $700,000 advertising campaign this year "to enhance the image of
doctors and to defeat 'the more radical national health insurance proposals' in
Congress".[54] Individual hospitals, and the American Hospital Association
(AHA), have been sponsoring newspaper advertisements designed to answer
the charge that hospitals are at the heart of the cost crisis, a charge that derives
from the fact that hospital costs account for almost 40 percent of the nation's
health care expenditures and are rising faster than other health care prices.
This situation led the Carter Administration last year to propose its controversial "cap" on hospital revenues and has pushed hospitals into a defensive
posture:

> We're seeing hospitals use advertising not to solicit, not to get new
> business, but as a defensive tool to tell their story. Hospitals all
> across the country are taking out ads explaining why costs have
> increased and how their products have changed. This is going to
> cause an unbelievable increase in hospital advertising.
>
> Michael D. Bromberg.

The campaign being sponsored by the AHA illustrates Bromberg's point.
Its message is summed up by this excerpt: "We think it's worth it . . . to make
hearts beat again, legs run again, eyes see again. For our profit and loss is
measured in lives. And we think that's the way you want it. Today's Hospital
Care—it's the bargain of your life."[55] This is powerful copy, but the most
arresting recent examples of "issues advertising" in health are probably the
AEtna ads, discussed by Lawton in part II. The insurance industry—more than
others in health—stands to lose a significant market should some of the
proposed national health insurance schemes become law. AEtna's campaign
seeks to portray the cost crisis as "systemic" and not the fault of any one
element of the system alone.

Some observers contend that the private insurance industry has been
remiss. For example, Stokes, in part II, advocates more effective communica-

tion to employees about their coverage under the benefit package and the choices open to them:

> *I recently completed a year-and-a-half-long project rewriting an old insurance plan into intelligible English. In doing that I gathered insurance booklets, HMO booklets, and the like from all over, looking for one that described plan coverage through an illustrative episode of illness—say appendicitis—from the first visit to the doctor through surgery and postoperative recovery. A comprehensive example like this would permit the employee to compare the coverage offered by various different insurance plans and HMOs. I found nothing of the kind. I don't know why this doesn't exist—it should. And the responsibility for this—or the opportunity—really belongs with the employer.*
>
> Linda K. Stokes

Insurance carriers could help employers put this kind of information together. One likely consequence of the *Bates* decision and the FTC activities in health will be an increase in the amount and sophistication of information available on physicians' fees. As this occurs, employers and union leaders may decide that disseminating information about differential physician fees in the community is in their own best interest and that of their employees or members, whether or not their health insurance plans include direct cost-sharing provisions, such as copayment and deductibles.

The Future: Professionalism, Commercialism, and Consumerism—Where Do the Scales Tip?

Until the FTC investigations have run their full course, no one can predict with certainty what the rules governing health professional advertising will be, much less what effect they will have. Still, some are willing to offer informed professional opinions on the two immediate questions that arise. First, how much and what kind of advertising is likely to be permitted and to take place, and second, what will relaxed rules on physician advertising mean for fees and costs of care? The persistent longer range question is what impact—positive and negative—can all this be expected to have on the quality of health care.

The Kinds of Advertising Anticipated

Truth will be the ultimate test for physicians—as for all advertisers— and, as in the general case, fixing standards of truth will be difficult. Whatever the FTC investigations may establish concerning the appropriate avenue to enforcement of standards, some rules of thumb will no doubt emerge to help

PHYSICIAN ADVERTISING: SOLICITATION OR INFORMATION?

Claude E. Welch: I see only one reason to advertise, and that is to sell a product. The Texas licensing board states that if a physician puts a statement in a paper for six days it's advertising, but on the seventh it becomes solicitation. When you get down to the nitty gritty, it becomes very difficult to know which is which. Somebody's going to have to adjudicate that, and I can see the state medical boards with a big job unless we're careful about what it is we are unleashing.

Emlyn I. Griffith: There is no simple answer, but I think the thrust of professional advertising should not be solicitation or self-laudation, but dissemination of relevant information and assistance to the public in making informed choices. The crux of the issue is what's the primary intent of professional advertising. We delude ourselves if we say that there isn't some self-serving in all advertising, some element of solicitation. By the same token, there is an element of solicitation in any kind of professional activity; we can't eliminate it. We have to concentrate on the principal objective, which is serving the public, furnishing information to the public about the availability of professional services.

Sol Levine: Various kinds of aesthetic concerns and questions of propriety lie just below the surface here. There are professional considerations, of course, and some strong economic concerns, but I believe there are a number of physicians whose prestige is firmly established and who don't worry about economic consequences of advertising, who are assured, always, of very good fees, who nevertheless are deeply concerned about certain kinds of advertising and solicitation as not being appropriate and proper. The sanctity of the profession seems to be at issue to some and many indeed see the doctor-patient relationship as a kind of sacred trust that could be violated, in a sense, by advertising. They do not like the prospect of seeing physicians involved in soliciting customers as tradespeople do.

Robert L. Biblo: We are kidding ourselves if we fail to look at this in terms of today, this world, this reality. There are situations now that didn't exist not so long ago. In urban centers and desirable places to live, there are lots of physicians. We seldom talk about how physicians *do* fight for patients. It is not very professional, so it doesn't become public, but physicians certainly do solicit patients and vie for referrals.

Morris E. Chafetz: My colleagues in medicine would not think ill of me if, in the event I moved back to Boston, I printed up a card with my name, address, and specialty and sent it to the physicians in town. That's perfectly legitimate; it is done all the time. They would think: "Isn't that nice, when we have something we are too busy to do ourselves, we will throw him a bone if he behaves himself." But suppose I'm an eager beaver. Why shouldn't I take that tasteful, low key announcement that no one minds my sending to my colleagues and instead place it in the *Boston Globe* and pay envelopes that are distributed around town? What is so wrong about that?

Lawrence K. Altman: Subtle forms of advertising, if not labeled as such, go on all the time—reports in medical journals that find their way into press releases and into the media. Teaching hospitals and large medical centers generate considerable publicity through such public relations activities. Even want ads can be a kind of institutional advertisement. Whether that's good or bad is not the issue. We should think about this in discussing questions like who can afford to advertise where, how often, and at how much cost.

Clark C. Havighurst: This examination of the benefits and risks of allowing solicitation needs to be examined rather carefully, because, put in a legal framework, it doesn't hold up well—indeed, it isn't relevant. Physician advertising comes up in two legal contexts—constitutional law, which applies to legislatures and state administrative bodies, and antitrust law, which applies to collective private action—in this instance, through medical societies. Both the Constitution and the Sherman Act are refreshingly antipaternalistic in their essential notions: both rest in part on the assumption that the citizen-consumer knows best. To say that the providers of medical services should be allowed to protect consumers from the hazards to which they might be subjected if advertising were widespread is quite at odds with the premise of both the antitrust laws and the First Amendment. It is another way of saying that citizens can't be trusted with information and that competition is not acceptable in the medical industry, and I think the profession may find it necessary to amend both the Constitution and the antitrust laws in order to establish those propositions as public policy.

Christopher Lovelock: I believe we should distinguish between factual information and what I call persuasive communication. When we think of advertising today we tend to think only of persuasion, but a great deal of paid media advertising is in fact simply provision of facts. We need to draw a careful distinction between a provider's efforts to persuade consumers that his services are better than those of the guy down the street, on the one hand, and provision of information about expertise, with some kind of outside evaluation of the types of services being provided, and how consumers react to it. I believe there is a danger in persuasive communications undertaken by one individual. I think the answer is to somehow have the information evaluated by a responsible independent group—and by independent, I mean independent of practitioners.

define truth in health professional advertising and the boundaries of fraud and deception.

The AMA draws its line at solicitation: information is ethical; solicitation is not. But as the quotations in the box attest, defining solicitation is itself a subjective exercise because the question reduces finally to the advertiser's *intent*. It may be more productive to focus instead on the advertisement's effect.

Surely an advertisement is deceptive if it contains wrong information or half-truths that mislead and create false expectations. "I can cure cancer for $10" falls easily into this category. Less obvious is a claim like "abdominal problems treated without surgery," which the AMA cites in its brief for the FTC to illustrate the dilemma of advertising that may be true but misleading:

> This sort of claim, even if true, exposes the consumer to the treacheries of the quack and bait-and-switch advertiser. The consumer, anxious about the potential seriousness of disquieting conditions and eager to avoid the pain and risks associated with surgery, is often most vulnerable to promises of quick cures, painless remedies, or medically unjustified hopes held out by a practitioner who has not even conducted an individual examination.[56]

One basic test is whether the claim can be verified:

> *I suggest the following two simple rules: first, does the ad contain verifiable facts and, second, is there anything in it that the resourceful prospective patient couldn't find if he worked hard enough at it. Beyond that I think it should be up to the advertiser to put in what he wants, so long as it's truthful and verifiable.*
> Gregory J. Ahart

Ahart's rules preclude puffery and self-aggrandizing claims like "I'm the best, or cheapest, plastic surgeon in town." Testimonials may be misleading because they stress irrelevant information; a sample of one hardly makes the general case. Illustrative of this is an actual advertisement that was reproduced in a *Newsweek* article on physician advertising: "I Did It! I answered this ad—80 lbs. ago—went from size 44 pants to my ideal size 7–8. I'm so grateful to be on Dr. Julian's program. Sincerely, Genevieve Fitzmaurice, R.N."[57] So long as Nurse Fitzmaurice really did lose eighty pounds (like Bruce Jenner and his Wheaties), and so long as she was enrolled as a participant in Dr. Julian's program, the advertisement is technically truthful because who is to say whether the program caused the weight reduction? In its brief before the FTC, the AMA expressed concern that testimonials of this nature would mislead consumers. But the courts have usually held that while truth in advertising should be regulated, relevance may be left to the consumer's judgment.[58] Whether the medical consumer will be judged especially in need of the law's protection remains to be seen.

Another thorny issue is fee advertising. The dissenting justices in the *Bates* case expressed misgivings, and some physicians argue that wide variations in fees make any kind of fee advertising inherently deceptive:

*There are no routine fees in medicine really. The human being
cannot be put on an assembly line and never will.*

George R. Dunlop

Dunlop's assertion is seriously challenged, however, by several practical facts:
the existence of relative value scales for some procedures, the ability of most
group practices and many solo practitioners to standardize their fees for certain
routine services, and the apparent ease with which physicians and hospitals
were able to comply with the government's requirement that they post their
base fees during the period of wage and price controls from 1971 to 1974.
Business Week reported in December 1971: the Price Commission "has
injected itself into high medical politics through its requirement that physicians as well as hospitals act like other retailers and post base prices and
subsequent increases prominently in their places of business . . . And the AMA
has accepted the posting provision without a qualm."[59]

Simplification—an essential technique of advertising—can itself create
deception:

> *If you're going to provide information that's meaningful, it should
> be total information. One of the problems that arises in talking
> about physicians' fees is that the fee does not represent what the
> total cost of the illness will be. We should be looking for responsi-
> ble ways of providing information on the range of cost for a total
> episode of illness.*

H. Frank Newman

Newman's proposal resembles the year-and-a-half project Stokes undertook.
The possibility of requiring certain kinds of disclosure can be carried several
steps farther, as the quotations in the box suggest. Those who advocate mandatory disclosure admit potential problems with legalities or practicability. But
they do suggest, as did the Supreme Court in *Bates*, that appropriate preventive
measures can be taken against harmful advertising, indeed that widely available information may itself be the best protection, if it stimulates discussion and
clarification. If advertising by individual practitioners were openly permitted,
the AMA and other concerned groups might be inspired to run counteradver-
tisements raising publicly some of the concerns voiced to the FTC and alerting
consumers to potential pitfalls. An approach like this would be consistent with
the professional ideals of self-regulation and protection of the public interest
and might be an important contribution to improved health education.

How much advertising physicians will elect to do in the absence of any
restraints is a separate question from how much they will be permitted to do, or
conversely, how much organized medicine will be allowed to restrain. Some
six months after the *Bates* case, preliminary indications suggest that few
physicians were eagerly awaiting that decision, advertising copy in hand:

> *An important question is what has happened in practice in New
> York since October when the Regents' decision took effect. From
> what I can piece together, the answer seems to be that there have*

FROM VOLUNTARY TO MANDATORY DISCLOSURE—AND BACK

Robert D. Reinecke: Granted that the public needs more information, which we all seem prepared to admit, why not require physicians and HMOs to advertise specific aspects of their services at certain intervals? This might get around this disturbing problem that advertising will be uneven and self-serving, and instead really fill a need.

Michael Lawson: I think that would be a serious mistake. The point is that we don't know what kind of advertising is going to be used and we don't know what effect it would have on the health care delivery system. Mandating it would be precipitious and unwise.

Clark C. Havighurst: The kind of regulation of advertising which seems most likely to stand up in court, and which might meet some of the needs that consumers have for information, would require mandatory disclosure of clarifying information if certain items are mentioned. For example, if you advertise price, you must state that additional services may be billed for. Drug advertising is subject to such regulation—a lot of fine print about risks and side effects must be provided with the ads.

George J. Annas: There is going to be a lot of data shortly available to a lot of people. I would suggest that as much as we might like to control it, we are probably not going to be able to and probably the best thing to do is just let the data out and let everyone comment on it and give their qualifications for commenting.

Paul M. Gertman: I'd like to propose a challenge experiment. Suppose we allow a physician to advertise anything he wants to on the condition that he agrees to permit access to his personally identifiable PSRO files, complaint files at the Board of Registration, and so on. This way people could verify his claims and the consumer would be protected from fraud.

Willis B. Goldbeck: Let's turn this question around for a minute and ask what physicians can do for advertising instead of what advertising can do for physicians. This is a concern of industry. If the real issue in physician advertising is protecting the public, shouldn't the medical societies be joining with the few "radicals" who would like to see the elimination of all unhealthful advertising? A very high percentage of television food commercials promote products that are high in saturated fat, cholesterol, sugar, or salt. And what about cigarette and alcohol advertising? Maybe that's where our information embargo ought to be placed, if it's the public health interest we're after.

been very few ads. We've been assuming that advertising is here and that the public wants it. But is that true? Is there really a demand? Is it an idea only consumer elites believe necessary or could it be something whose time has not yet come?

Lawrence K. Altman

Certainly it is too early to draw firm conclusions either way. The *Bates* decision has not definitively laid to rest doubts about the propriety or even the legality of all physician advertising. State laws prohibiting physician advertising exist in ten states, and only four leave physician advertising completely unregulated.[60] Even had the court removed all uncertainty, Paul N. Bloom believes some lag in advertising would occur simply because old habits die slowly:

There's been so little advertising because collusion has gone on for so long, and suddenly is declared illegal. Physicians are still wary and watching one another. Also, advertising is expensive, especially in the New York area, and people are going to have to find efficient mechanisms—community newspapers, direct mail, and so on. When they find the mechanism and figure out what kinds of information consumers will use, then we will see advertising, but it will take time.

Perhaps rather than habit, reluctance to advertise may reflect an astute reading of the public mind:

The reason we haven't seen many ads is that doctors are seasoned marketers and they've made the correct judgment that advertising is not the way to build a practice today. I'm all for advertising, but it's my hunch that the public isn't ready yet and won't be for some five to twenty years or so. The physicians who lead the way in this may have a very rough time.

Robert F. Froehlke

What Effect on Fees and Costs?

Implicit in the FTC's interest in physician advertising is the conviction that fees and costs are artificially high in the absence of competitive pressures and would be lowered if more advertising were done. Based more on theory than on empirical evidence, the case can be argued both ways. Third-party payment is a negative consideration:

The fact is that most people don't pay fees directly. I question what, if any, impact fee advertising will have on selecting physicians or hospitals when most of the fees are being paid by someone else.

Arthur G. Carty

On the positive side, fee advertising should spotlight fees that are out of line and maybe force them down, or stabilize fees at present levels and restrain major increases. It also seems logical that some services—those that are more discretionary and more often financed out-of-pocket—would show some price elasticity if advertised openly.

Of particular concern is the danger that physician advertising would stimulate substantial new demand—false demand—for health services:

> As we have more and more pediatricians and fewer kids, three things will probably happen. Pediatricians will start arguing that they should care for older kids, they'll start threatening family practice and call themselves family pediatricians, and they'll define new morbidity. These are market phenomena, and as we talk about fees and prices we should bear in mind that aggregate costs are strongly influenced by such forces.
>
> Rick J. Carlson

How efficiently physicians induce demand for health care is a major research question in economics. As yet, it remains a puzzle, but in highly discretionary procedures there is probably valid cause for concern.

> I fear that a great many people will be persuaded by advertising to have their noses pulled down or lifted just a bit. Any way you look at it, advertising is sure to be inflationary.
>
> Claude E. Welch

Until more data are available, the cost picture will remain muddled. Fee advertising by physicians would probably raise the advertiser's cost of doing business and might generate some extra demand for services, but might also reduce consumers' search costs and elevate their consciousness of price:

> Bringing physicians' fees out into the open is important but it won't be a panacea. It is, however, a necessary first step to encouraging people to feel that it's O.K. to ask a doctor about his fees.
>
> Robert D. Reinecke

Compounding the confusion, consumer awareness of price could conceivably cut both ways:

> Unfortunately, what I see in my practice is that the best advertisement for a doctor around Boston is to have higher fees. Patients of all income levels feel that if he is expensive he must be good. I think most doctors get more return on their "advertising" dollar by investing in Brooks Brothers suits and a nicely decorated office than by putting something in the newspaper.
>
> Warren Kantrowitz

On balance, the impact of advertising on health care costs may be subordinate to other considerations, in particular, the general question of how much value the dollars are returning.

What Relationship to Quality?

Once the utility of publicizing at least some information on physicians' fees is granted, the clash over advertising reduces to starkly conflicting views of the appropriate measures of quality in health care and whose role it is to define and enforce them:

> The culture of medicine is somewhat threatened by these pressures for fuller information. Not only is fee-for-service being questioned, but so is the basic precept that only a physician's peers are qualified to evaluate his work. There are various movements in our society encouraging consumers to question whether professionals are the only ones to make these determinations.
>
> Sol Levine

The "movements" Levine alludes to, together with a highly publicized "malpractice crisis" and government-mandated performance review programs for the care of publicly subsidized patients, have intensified interest in the quality of care and undermined confidence in the traditional approach to assuring quality strictly through personnel licensure with an overlay of continuing medical education. State licensing boards control entry into the health professions and theoretically assure the uninformed consumer that the licensed physician, dentist, nurse, pharmacist, or other practitioner has attained a minimal level of competence. However, these boards seldom resort to disciplinary measures[61] and a feeling has grown that the profession's self-policing may be inadequate, whether looking in from the outside:

> It has been said that physicians have a well-developed set of professional standards to go by, but there's one major problem. The consumer/patient doesn't know what the standards are, so from the consumer's point of view they're irrelevant. If the public were more aware of the numbers of procedures that are considered optimal to keep a surgeon's skill finely tuned, for example, then the consumer could begin to apply those standards and look for deviations. The value of those standards from the standpoint of communication is very low right now because only one side of the communication process knows what the standard is.
>
> Willis B. Goldbeck

or welling up from within:

> I'll accept on faith that all the structures of medicine—medical societies, peer review, college of surgeons, boards and all that—are absolutely concerned and dedicated to protecting the public against the malpractitioner. Even if our intentions are noble and right, I think we have to take into account that a greater informed public questions our motives, sees in these structures a guild situation used by those in power to perpetuate monopoly. Saccharin is a case in point. The scientific community, measuring Canadian rats, said in its wisdom that saccharin was a carcinogenic agent. The public put up such a row that Congress had to

THE QUALITY CONUNDRUM: "BATTING AVERAGES," PRACTICE PATTERNS, AND THE ROLE OF CONSUMER PREFERENCES

Paul M. Gertman: PSROs are now generating a lot of data on physician qualifications and experiences—who's done a particular surgical procedure, how often, and with what complication rates, etc. There is now opposition to release of that data, but I believe over the next decade we're going to have to come to grips with opening it up.

Claude E. Welch: I regret very much if it has to go as far as Dr. Gertman suggests, because then if a surgeon hasn't taken out ten gall bladders in the last six months the next patient who comes through his office door with a pain in the abdomen might be in a good deal of trouble. The need to fill that quota, so to speak, might get in the way of objectivity. And that would be reprehensible.

George J. Annas: It's tough to know what types of information— batting averages, success rates—the public should be privy to because the data are difficult to interpret. No doubt about that. My own bias, however, is to give the public all the information that is reasonably available to professionals making decisions. Surgeons have unwritten criteria they use to evaluate colleagues when they are referring patients or friends or family—facts like how often he's doing the procedure and how successfully. That is the kind of hard data the public should have.

Robert D. Reinecke: It's a naive assumption, I believe, that the public and even the medical profession would use such information if it were available. I submit that most of you would not know how to evaluate outcomes data, say, on eye surgery, and even if you did, wouldn't bother but would continue to use the same informal communication channels you now use.

Morris E. Chafetz: This "batting average" suggestion may have been facetious, but I find it intriguing. Maybe a bunch of health professionals ought to gather together a conference and try to hammer out how we might establish a batting average that would have some meaning to ourselves and the public.

Dr. Welch: I don't share this worry about being unable to tell whether a doctor is a good doctor. Peer review is the only way to do it. We have licensure, specialty boards of the AMA which are an extremely good indicator in general terms of the adequacy of a physician's education, and also membership in some of the professional societies, continuing medical education, hospital privileges, and so on. These won't hold in every individual case, but in general they are good indices.

Robert F. Froehlke: Today society is not going to accept any profession, including the medical profession, policing itself. Sure, the medical profession is capable of determining quality. But now the public should have the facts needed to begin making their own judgments.

Christopher Lovelock: We should think in terms of generating consumer evaluations of health services and of developing mechanisms for providing a fair and reasonable way of finding out what consumers prefer.

Elizabeth M. Kurella: There is going to be a lot more input on the part of patients as to what they want. Some will choose a paternalistic doctor who will take care of everything for them; others will make different choices to suit their needs and predilections. I think people are going to demand enough information to make those discriminations for themselves.

Russell B. Roth: "Consumer satisfaction" talk disturbs me. Many a physician has built up a great practice by developing his bedside manner as a substitute for professional competence. When I've been involved in efforts of the profession to police itself and deal with mountebanks and charlatans, I have never seen a case go to trial without a line-up of satisfied patients giving enthusiastic character references and telling how much good the doctor did for them. Consumer satisfaction is a fascinating thing to analyze.

John I. Sandson: I am hearing too much talk here about technical aspects of surgery and almost nothing about the problem we've been struggling with in medical education—how to get the art back into medicine. It is difficult to measure so it gets shunted aside, but it is an awfully big part of the practice of medicine.

Sol Levine: I'd like to pick up on that and suggest—not facetiously at all, but respectfully: Would it not be appropriate for a physician to provide the following types of information: "I provide health education, I spend a good deal of time discussing how people can adhere to medical regimens. I answer questions and regard them as very important. I try not to overbook—there's not much waiting time. My receptionist and nurse are well-trained and pleasant and so am I. I'm available weekends and I don't charge for telephone consultations." I think these are legitimate things that consumers want to know.

intervene. The point is that people are sick and tired of our paternalistic view that we know what's best for them. And if we want to get along we've got to try to listen to them because they're trying to tell us something.

Morris E. Chafetz

Consumers of health services need objective, evaluated, and accurate information they can trust. Advertising—by definition openly partisan—can hardly satisfy this need, but could possibly open the way for the kind of effort that seems widely regarded as promising:

We mustn't limit out thinking on quality to the outrageous malpractice cases where someone's made a dreadful mistake. Instead we should be thinking creatively in terms of consumer evaluations of health care services and how to develop fair and reasonable mechanisms for finding out how consumers feel about the services they receive. Physicians need to think of advertising and marketing not in the limited sense of persuading patients to select a particular practitioner but rather as an opportunity for providing information on what their expertise is, including some objective outside evaluation. So again I come back to the belief that we must begin by finding out what consumers want, and like, and think.

Christopher Lovelock

National health planning guidelines recently published[62] by the federal government attest to a growing concensus that standards of performance can and should be developed for the medical profession. The quotations in the box suggest measures to begin factoring the consumer's views into the quality equation and providing information consumers can evaluate and use. In a beginning, tentative way they suggest the direction we can move, in this arena of relaxed rules about physician advertising, toward the door behind which waits the lady, not the tiger.

Solicitation, HMOs, and Employee Choices

3

While the medical profession struggles with the possibility that medicine is really part "business," and necessarily entails subtle or even overt competition for patients, health maintenance organizations are forging ahead with a direct marketing approach. Competition among alternative delivery systems is the watchword of the "HMO strategy"; solicitation of members is a sine qua non.

The reasoning and a little of the history behind this development are the focus of this chapter. The first volume in this series described salient features of HMOs,[1] and the next volume will deal intensively with what is and is not known about what they can do and what they may mean for industry as payer for and provider of care. Taking off from the Department of Health, Education and Welfare's March 10, 1978, conference on industry and HMOs, that fifth volume in the series will define and illustrate the major HMO prototypes, examine and contrast the "track records" of some, and speculate on apparent prerequisites of success.

For now confining our attention to HMO features that reflect on information for employees' decisions about health, this chapter forms a bridge connecting organized medicine's rules on advertising to the theme of competition in health care and the employer's role in the employee's choice of a provider. The Health Maintenance Organization Act of 1973 affirmed the legality of advertising by qualified HMOs and gave them a "foot in the door" of potential employee markets. The impact of these two provisions will extend well beyond federally qualified HMOs, indeed could alter profoundly the marketplace for health.

HMOs and Organized Medicine: A Three Decade Duel

The Federal Trade Commission's current charges against the American Medical Association are considered the most serious the AMA has faced since its conviction in 1943 of a criminal antitrust conspiracy to restrain competition.[2] The bone of contention in that first serious skirmish was a prepaid health plan—the Group Health Association of Washington, D.C.—one of the nation's pioneering prepaid plans. Even before that, the Ross-Loos Medical Group, founded in 1929 by two Los Angeles physicians, had problems with the local medical establishment. Sensing in the new plan a threat to practices and incomes already eroded by the Great Depression, Los Angeles physicians strenuously objected to it, largely on grounds that it violated the patient's free choice of physician. In 1934 the county medical society expelled Drs. Ross and Loos, but the AMA Judicial Council overruled the local decision, in part to avert adverse publicity, and the two maverick physicians were reinstated.[3] The incident illustrates the profession's intense distrust of and opposition to prepaid plans from their inception.

Two decades passed before prepaid health plans began overcoming some of those early handicaps and convincing the public of their capacity to deliver good quality medical care at decreased cost,[4] by using almost 50 percent fewer hospital days.[5] The remaining history is well-known: Ellwood's "health maintenance strategy,"[6] complete with catchy new acronym; Nixon's 1971 health message to Congress launching the Federal HMO movement; and Congress' passage two years later of the Health Maintenance Organization Act of 1973 (P.L. 93–222), a piece of "enabling legislation" that created as many roadblocks as it removed.[7] Amendments passed in October 1976 (P.L. 94–640) addressed the problems inherent in the earlier statute, offered HMOs seeking federal qualification greater organizational flexibility, and extended through 1980 the original five-year development authority of the federal HMO program. This program, lodged in the Department of Health, Education, and Welfare (HEW), has been much criticized for lack of direction and a slow start.[8]

More recent history is more familiar still: endorsements of the HMO concept as a "centerpiece" of the Carter administration's cost containment policy, first by HEW Undersecretary Hale Champion, then by Secretary Joseph Califano, who convened the highly publicized March 10 meeting on HMOs for the nation's industrial and labor leaders. The recent executive branch attention to HMOs derives chiefly from concern over uncontrollable health care costs which seem to stand in the way of pursuing other policy objectives in health, particularly President Carter's campaign pledge of a national health insurance plan.

Two overlapping imperatives are driving the HMO movement. One is a pragmatic search for long-term solutions to the problem of health care costs. HMOs are seen as devices that can achieve economies by restructuring financial incentives on physicians to encourage appropriate use of high-cost hospital care and other discretionary services, along with peer review, management controls, and an appropriate manpower mix.

The second emphasizes solutions to the cost crisis that lean more heavily on the private sector than on increasingly tight regulations and movement toward a monolithic publicly managed system of care. HMOs are viewed as a key feature in the strategy to bring costs under control through a market-oriented approach. The emphasis is on restructuring the delivery system and reinstilling some elements of competition by challenging the unstructured fee-for-service solo practitioner to reexamine his own practice.

The broader market-oriented view is the more relevant to the topic at hand because availability of information is a necessary ingredient. The theory of market imperfections in health rests heavily on the notion of consumer ignorance, and most strategies to strengthen the market include efforts to improve the information available to consumers. The flaws in the medical market are now widely recognized—perverse incentives that foster inefficiency and indifference to costs, like the third-party payment scheme that removes price as a consideration through extensive frontend benefits and disproportionate coverage for hospital-based, high-technology procedures; the physician's control of demand through his ordering decisions for hospitalization, tests, and prescriptions; and the provider's possession of technical knowledge to which average consumers have little access. These and other factors are discussed more fully in the first volume of the series, which stresses that employment-related health insurance has been a major disincentive toward efficiency in the health market. The dilemma, of course, is that Americans like this protection. As a society we value medical care, and we want guaranteed access to it. Most of us would resist any significant reduction in our insurance coverage. And so we look for ways to maintain that financial protection while curbing its inflationary tendencies. Part of the HMO's appeal is that it seems to some extent to offer the best of both worlds—comprehensive coverage in a cost-efficient framework which operates in part by addressing the consumer's problem of finding a health care provider:

> We need information that allows for selection on the basis of criteria including costs, quality and access, peer review, and other elements that constitute cost-effective, quality care. I'm convinced that grouping of providers and prepayment of enrollees are the necessary mechanisms. Prepaid rate structures permit consumers to make their purchasing decisions about health care at a moment of untroubled analytical reflection, rather than at the moment of high anxiety when illness has struck.
>
> Geoffrey V. Heller

The HMO and Competition

Because they represent a closed system of care, offering a defined package of services to an enrolled population at a fixed price, HMOs invite comparisons with other available options on the basis of performance characteristics such as days of hospitalization per 1000 enrollees, annual costs per person, and other verifiable measures. That these comparisons challenge the status quo is attested to by this exchange between a surgeon and a psychiatrist:

> HMOs have built in some financial incentives to keep utilization down. That's the one thing that they have that the unstructured fee-for-service sector doesn't have. It's one of our great weaknesses and we're going to have to do something about it.
>
> George R. Dunlop

> This is the first time in my thirty years in the medicine that I've heard someone in a position of power in the medical establishment say "Let's look at how we might adapt to a changing situation." I think that's a crucial statement, and a very positive one.
>
> Morris E. Chafetz

The suggestion that HMOs can foster widespread and salutary competition for the health care dollar has intuitive appeal and confirmed adherents, although research evidence on the point is as yet scanty.[9,10,11] The most recent published study of the effects of HMOs on competition was issued by the Federal Trade Commission in July 1977. To test "the hypothesis that the presence of an HMO in an area can have a competitive impact upon the traditional fee-for-service sector," the study analyzed correlations in nine geographic areas between HMO market share and the hospital utilization rates and size of benefit packages of area Blue Cross plans. From statistical and qualitative observations, the FTC economists conclude that "a significant HMO presence may help lower costs not only to HMO subscribers but to others in the area, as well."[12]

A different kind of evidence of HMOs' competitive impact on the fee-for-service sector can be found in interactions between the two major types of HMO—the closed-panel prepaid group practice plan (PGP) and the open-panel, fee-for-service individual practice association (IPA). IPAs tend to emerge in areas where PGPs are either established or being planned; frequently, they represent self-defense on the part of area physicians faced with the perceived threat of a PGP—clearly a response to competitive pressures. IPAs that successfully hold down utilization and achieve significant economies[13] in turn challenge solo practitioners and the unorganized fee-for-service sector. At the end of 1977, there were some 165 HMOs of all descriptions in operation, with a combined enrollment of about 6.5 million, about 90 percent of which is PGP membership.[14] These numbers represent some growth in recent years. For example, there were only thirty-one operational HMOs in February 1971,[15] and HMO enrollment increased 10 percent in the six months preceding April 1975.[16] Still, HMO members constitute only about 3 percent of the total population. If HMOs are to have an appreciable impact, the rate of growth will have to accelerate rapidly in the very near future. The purpose of the 1973 HMO Act, the 1976 amendments, and recent government rhetoric is to provide the needed impetus to that growth. One of the government's chief inducements to HMO growth is the "dual choice" provision of the HMO Act.

The HMO and Employee Choices

Section 1310 of the HMO Act, as expounded in regulations and as amended, stipulates that each employer covered by the Fair Labor Standards Act (that is, subject to minimum wage laws) and employing twenty-five or more people must offer, as part of an existing health benefit plan, the option of membership in a federally qualified HMO, if available. Federally qualified plans have met standards concerning the legal and financial soundness of the plan and its willingness and capacity to provide the scope of services stipulated in federal regulations. If both a PGP and an IPA are qualified and available, one of each type must be offered, but if there is more than one of either type, the employer may begin to pick and choose among those available within each of the two categories.

The initiative to activate the dual choice option rests with the qualified HMO. It must file a written request, including specific information about the status and ownership of the plan, its service area, facilities, premium, and marketing material, at least 180 days before the expiration of the existing health benefits contract and 90 days before the expiration of the union contract, if applicable. The insinuation of mandatory dual choice to collective bargaining was hotly contested by unions who saw it as an encroachment on their bargaining "turf." Promulgation of the regulations implementing dual choice was delayed by this controversy, which was resolved finally by granting the unions' right to disapprove an HMO's petition for inclusion in a collectively bargained plan, whereupon the employer is absolved of further obligation with regard to that HMO's access to the collective bargaining unit.

The employer is not required to pay more in order to offer the HMO options; employees may ask the employer to deduct any incremental premium costs from their paychecks or they may collectively bargain for the difference. Originally, the employer was required to offer an HMO so long as it could claim one of his employees as a resident of its service area. The 1976 amendments recognized the administrative burden this placed on large and/or geographically dispersed firms, and adjusted the provision so that the HMO's service area must encompass the residences of at least twenty-five of the firm's employees to justify inclusion in the firm's health benefits program.

These dual choice stipulations, although painstakingly specific, leave the employer a wide band of discretion, especially vis-à-vis HMOs that are not federally qualified. By mandating that employers interact with federally qualified HMOs that approach them, the HMO Act may encourage some in industry to look more closely at all HMOs and at the health care delivery system to which employee benefit plans are the financial access route. This raises new questions about relationships between benefit plans and medical services, areas heretofore often compartmentalized in corporate structures and thinking. The dual choice mandate adds a new dimension to the health benefit plan, by returning to the employee a major decision concerning his coverage, and also by enlarging the role of the employer and the union. With the obligation to present options to employees comes the responsibility—and the opportunity, as posited by Stokes in part II—to begin fostering a fuller appreciation of the scope of the health benefit package, its dollar value compared with available alternatives, and the appropriate and inappropriate uses of medical care services.

The dual choice provision also makes the employer or union a gatekeeper, with the authority to choose which of several HMOs best represent the alternatives open to employees. Some employers offer more different HMO options that the law requires or include HMO options in areas where none are federally qualified. For example, a May 1975 study conducted before the promulgation of the dual choice regulations found that 19 percent of the 300 large corporations surveyed already offered a dual choice option and another 3 percent were "working on it."[17]

The first volume of this series described industry's "continuous but variable" involvement in the half-century history of prepaid health plans and suggested that impressive HMO penetration of employee markets has been largely confined to HMO strongholds—places like San Francisco, indeed all of California, Rochester, Minneapolis–St. Paul, and Washington, D.C. Elsewhere, some employers report desultory responses to conscientious enrollment drives and sometimes express deep concern that the HMO concept is being oversold. Lack of enthusiasm for the HMO option may reflect the employee group's unfamiliarity with the concept, satisfaction with the existing benefit package and with established providers, or simple inertia. The effective HMOs recognize that their marketing strategies are critical. They are acutely aware of the hazard of overselling.

Some Industry Reservations about HMOs

Literature on marketing HMOs almost invariably characterizes mandatory dual choice as a final resort, and even then probably futile in the absence of an appealing service package. HMOs are counseled to emphasize coordinated care, budgetable expenses, "one-stop shopping," possibly a more comprehensive range of benefits than the traditional insurance option, and better continuity of care for nearly equivalent premiums. Programs with monthly family premiums more than $10 or $15 higher than the alternative benefit package seldom achieve significant penetration, with or without mandatory dual choice.

On the industry side, insurance carriers and consultants, corporations and unions have developed various rules of thumb and checklists to guide employers in assessing an HMO. Because federal qualification cannot guarantee uniformly high-quality service, employers are counseled to take pains to assess the options being offered their employees:

Our role as consulting actuaries is to advise the corporate consumer on the subject of HMOs. One of the things we put up front is the problem of credibility. We warn our clients to evaluate the marketing claims of HMOs very carefully because we find that their marketing is often the least reliable guide to a realistic evaluation of their services.

Harold Gilbert

Caution is counseled because the employer's offer of membership in an HMO goes beyond mere insurance coverage to encompass a service package as well—an important distinction:

When offering an HMO, the employer is more on the line: he is no longer recommending just a health insurance option; he's now also recommending a medical care option and putting an imprimatur on it. Therefore, the prudent employer will be more critical in evaluating the Harvard Plan than, for example, Blue Cross/Blue Shield.

Robert S. Lurie

The Harvard Community Health Plan in metropolitan Boston, whose marketing history Lurie and Biblo trace in part II, is now firmly established with a secure reputation. The paper reveals that this was not always so and admits of early problems with overselling the product by establishing patterns of service that were impossible to sustain over the long haul. In addition, Biblo points out another challenge to HMO credibility—a sort of double standard with which they have to live:

Members of prepaid group practices make demands on the plan that they would not normally make of a medical care provider. People say of a traditional physician, "My doctor is so good, he kept me waiting for an hour before I could see him or it took me weeks to get an appointment." In a prepaid practice it's just the opposite. They tear the roof down if they have to wait. Members feel that they own the program and they bring different expectations. We try to tailor the program to meet those but we don't always succeed. And some of the demands placed on us are unreasonable or are related to some overselling we may have been guilty of at one time.

Robert L. Biblo

Undoubtedly, the worst rash of oversalesmanship of HMOs occurred in California in the early 1970s when the state decided to contract preferentially with prepaid plans for the care of public assistance recipients. This innovation was highly touted but fell "so far short of its promise that many consider it scandalous."[18] Some dismiss that unfortunate chapter in HMO history as an aberration best forgotten:

Coming from California, I frequently run into the question of what there is to be learned from the deviant HMO-like creatures that experimented under the state's Medicaid program. I would ask your indulgence to leave them out of the debate because I believe they did the whole HMO movement an unfair disservice. And they are not the California experience. The California experience is far more the very impressive record of the Kaiser Plan, Ross-Loos, the San Joaquin Foundation, and others.

Geoffrey V. Heller

But important lessons can be drawn from the Medi-Cal prepaid health plan experiments. They demonstrated the danger inherent in setting up a separate system of care for the poor and the limitations of competition as a guarantor of minimal quality, even of the nontechnical indices of quality that consumers can evaluate:

Once upon a time people naively believed that simply because the HMO would have to compete for patients, it would have to serve them well or lose them all a year or two later as a result of bad word-of-mouth. The unfortunate experience in California demonstrated that you could make a lot of money in those two years and retire very happily. What happened, in retrospect, probably shouldn't be very surprising—but I don't think we'll see it happen again.

John Friedland

As Friedland suggests, the California Medi-Cal experience also raises issues related to the role of private enterprise in HMO development. It is true that some of the California plans made excessive profits at the expense of quality, but it is also true that proprietary enterprises in health often deliver excellent care. And the stimulus private enterprise could provide may be essential to rapid growth of HMOs. Entrepreneurs can be expected to push the margins and challenge the assumptions that define acceptable bounds on marketing, advertising, and promotion:

We certainly need to enlist entrepreneurial instincts in developing HMOs rapidly. The private sector has been reluctant to plunge into HMO investment because at every stage since the idea became popular around 1970, there's been tremendous uncertainty about its future—all attributable to the government. We're always waiting—even now—for Congress or HEW to produce some definitive rules. That kind of uncertainty is not conducive to private development, and it's troubling but true that we seem unable to cure it.

Clark C. Havighurst

You're right about the climate. I think the proprietary hospital industry is going to view HMOs as a management opportunity rather than an investment opportunity, at least for the short term. The government says they're all for HMOs now and that the time is right, but we've heard them say that before. We may get involved as management consultants—just as we're now doing with nonprofit

*hospitals—but I see no sign of substantial short-term investment
until that cloud has lifted.*

Michael D. Bromberg

The HMO and Advertising

Even without entrepreneurial pressures, the margins of acceptable advertising are wider for HMOs than they are for the individual practitioner. Section
1311 of the HMO Act overrules state laws preventing a federally qualified HMO
from soliciting members "through advertising of services, charges or other
non-professional aspects of its operation." The statute defers to medical ethics
and "does not authorize any advertising which identifies or refers to or makes
any qualitative judgment concerning any health professional who provides
services to that HMO." A favorite challenge voiced by physicians antipathetic
to HMOs is that they be required to "play by the same rules" as the private
practitioner, in the name of fairness. But the traditional rules simply do not
apply to HMOs, which are relatively larger-scale enterprises and need to
advertise in order to get started and generate sufficient volume to achieve
economies of scale.[19]

The federal statute probably has less direct impact on HMO behavior than
do local customs and norms, as Biblo suggests is the case in the Boston area:

*The Harvard Plan talks about location, hours, and services—
straight information. We've not gone to radio and television
because our physicians find that too objectionable. The views of
the ethics committees of the local medical societies have changed
to permit taseful advertising, although local societies will criticize
us sometimes and have done so recently. But we have to concern
ourselves with our own physicians' views. And they have serious
doubts from their training concerning the ethics of advertising.*

Just as the constraints on solicitation are most onerous for a physician
trying to become established in a new location, advertising is especially
important to a new HMO in town:

*When you're starting out and you're an unknown entity, you have
to find ways to get people to look at your product. You have to find
the pioneer who's going to try it out.*

Robert L. Biblo

Research into the diffusion of innovation shows that the pioneer's decision is greatly facilitated and others are more willing to follow suit if the
general atmosphere is favorable.[20] Use of the mass media can help create such a
milieu, and Biblo feels that paid advertising, rather than the public relations
activities usually undertaken by nonprofit organizations, affords greater
control:

Public relations approaches leave you at the mercy of the individual journalist. Advertising allows you to reach large numbers of people and provide your own information.

Advertising is generally acknowledged as important, but there is no master template for launching a new HMO. The substance of the message depends on the HMO's situation, which varies according to environmental factors:

PLAYING THE PERCENTAGES: HOW MUCH DO THEY MEAN?

Robert L. Biblo: We're wrestling with the idea of providing more specific information in our ads—that is, if an organization such as the Harvard Plan hospitalizes half that of the state average, perhaps we should begin to say that in the public media, and give the reasons for it.

R. Hopkins Holmberg: Colleagues often migrate to my office with their Blue Cross option and their Harvard Community Health Plan option, looking for some guidance in their choice. They have very little information before them except a premium difference of a few dollars a month—nothing significant. The moment you say to them: "You know, we're not publishing this and it's not confirmed but my best indication is that your probability of being cut with a surgeon's knife is more than twice as great if you elect Blue Cross-and your probability of being hospitalized and out of work is twice as great," that affects them. That's information they want to hear. As employers we ought to be impressed by that too—in terms of absenteeism. In fact, I think we're being irresponsible in not making that information available.

Russell B. Roth: I train people to operate. And it so happens that two of the residents we've trained are urologists in qualified HMOs at present. I see them from time to time and I'm interested in this, so I ask them: "What is it that you do that I didn't teach you or what don't you do that I did teach you? What's the difference in the indication for prostectomy? Why do you do half as many?" Fewer procedures are being done and the question arises, is this good or is this bad? It's my strong suspicion that to evaluate this thing in terms of outcomes, we're going to have to study it for at least twenty more years.

I've been involved in the marketing of four or five HMO programs in Massachusetts and was in on the early discussions, going back to 1966, of the Harvard Community Health Plan. The most striking lesson from those experiences is that there isn't one way to go about it. The support, geography, industrial market, hospital configuration, and physician community are all factors. There may be a set of general rules, but the marketing and advertising problems are always significantly different.

Arthur G. Carty

John A. McLaren: From a marketing standpoint, this kind of information could have a negative impact, especially since it raises the question of whether the quality of the service in the HMO is as good as can be obtained elsewhere. We all hear stories about England under the national health service, where you wait for upwards of a year and a half for surgery. I think HMOs are sensitive to the risks of making known the amount of surgery, the amount of testing, and the amount of consultation they are avoiding.

Harold Gilbert: As an actuary I'm involved with statistics, and the occasional misleading use of them, so I'll identify my prejudice first. I'm firmly convinced that putting financial incentives on physicians definitely reduces the incidence of surgery and hospitalization. But I think the total disclosure of crude information like this could be grossly misleading, without careful qualification of limiting factors—the characteristics of the population involved, the choices available, and so on. I suggest that the only final criterion has to be: does the material mislead, not does it meet some preconceived standard of information to be disseminated. It's a difficult criterion to apply objectively, but I'm at a loss for a better one.

Alasdair C. MacIntyre: The problem of surgery has to be seen in statistical terms. Only then does one begin to come to grips with the dilemma of error in medicine. What has most alarmed me in public discussions of unnecessary surgery is that nobody comes straight out and says: if for a wide range of types of cases you perform surgery only on those who certainly need it, then a sizeable number who need the surgery won't get it. But if you perform enough surgery to make sure that everybody who needs it gets it, you will perform a large number of operations that are unnecessary for the people who have them.

And, to the degree possible, the situation of the target audience is part of the strategy:

> Marketers look for leverage points. They understand when consumers do things and why. Consumers actually make very few decisions about health care. A vast amount of decision making takes place when a person takes a new job—that's a high leverage point—you walk on your job, you move into a new town, what decision making information do you have: often only a brochure on health care. Several studies have shown that people find their doctors in the first six to eight weeks. That's the time to approach them with innovative approaches to health care delivery.
>
> Ronald Stiff

The marketing strategy also reflects the HMO's developmental stage. Having broken even and established an equilibrium within the community, for example, the Harvard Community Health Plan is debating how far it should now push its advertising message. The quotations in the box push much farther than the Harvard Plan seems likely to move in the foreseeable future, but they adumbrate a direction an aggressive campaign could logically take. They also crystallize several policy issues raised by HMO advertising: What kind of advertising will foster the maximum competition possible, and invite comparisons without misleading or deceiving consumers? What kinds of quality claims are advisable and appropriate for the HMO, and possible for the consumer to substantiate? To what extent can advertising promote, among alternative systems of care, a competitive health system that selects for quality and cost efficiency?

> Dr. Roth and Dr. Dunlop have both said, in different contexts, that we need to do very careful evaluations before we rush ahead and change things. They're right, of course, and we should also be asking of delivery systems the same tough questions they're asking about clinical medicine. We should be evaluating forms of health care—individual practitioners, neighborhood health centers, HMOs. We need a dialogue about the various alternatives, in which disparate viewpoints and positions are heard and an objective moderator makes certain that each side has its say, pro and con. Only then, I think, will we have some degree of confidence. HMOs are great for some people, no doubt, but they're probably not right for everyone, any more than the traditional doctor's office is right for everyone today.
>
> Christopher Lovelock

Much like the consumer-compiled physician directories discussed in chapter 2, Lovelock's quasi referendum is a means of bringing the patient's preferences into the collection, analysis, and presentation of information about alternative systems. But a distinction needs to be made between the aspects of quality that have much to do with consumer perception—things like accessibility of various sorts, responsiveness, and aspects that are more difficult for consumers to judge, perhaps because they occur infrequently and cannot be evaluated through personal experience or because they are highly technical.[21] Minimal standards in these spheres are set by licensure and credentialing regulations and authorities, but they leave above the threshold ample room for significant variation.

Even the technical aspects of quality in competing delivery systems may be susceptible to much more effective comparisons than are currently being made:

> Those of us who do quality-of-care research think it technically feasible to explicitly compare the quality of care between alternative delivery systems. We have a large number of standards and short-term outcome measures. You can compare any two large systems, which can accumulate 100,000 patient-years of experience. We can measure quite precisely comparative health care quality in those two large systems. I want to know who wants that information? We cannot identify a constituency for that type of research analysis.
>
> Paul M. Gertman

The impetus for the research would seem to have to come either from the system of care that believes it has the competitive edge, from the government or other large-scale payers for care interested in prudent purchases, or from inquiring consumer groups who, perhaps most of all, have a legitimate need to know:

> Clearly, the consumer, the worker, the public, you and I, have no hope of knowing the complexities of many issues that concern us. We want to know the "bottom line"—what does it mean—profit or loss; bargain or rip-off; safe or unsafe; wise or unwise. We, therefore, require evaluated information from a source, or preferably sources, that we are prepared to trust. Trust—there is the rub.[22]

Occupational Health Hazards: Management and Labor in a Vital Interaction

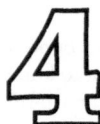

Occupational health hazards pose a separate set of problems from those related to finding a health care provider or selecting a system of care. At the ends of the spectrum, occupational health hazards are either acute and obvious, demanding nothing short of immediate and intense effort to remove them from the workplace, or entirely unsuspected, leaving little to be done. Between the two extremes lies a large and growing grey area that challenges traditional assumptions about roles and responsibilities in the interactions between management and labor. The wide middle of the spectrum is the focus of this chapter; the ambiguity of the risks makes effective communication vital—and difficult. Together with pressures created by the Occupational Safety and Health Act (OSHAct) of 1970 and with scientific findings at the tip of a possibly massive iceberg, the social movements toward self-determination discussed in the previous three chapters are accelerating demands within industry for better communication about occupational health hazards.

The occupational health problem is doubly complex. It involves not only a moving target—changing industrial processes that bring new substances into the workplace almost daily—but also an evolving and unpredictable arsenal—a continually growing scientific base and refinement in techniques that tend to alter the definition of the nature and scope of the problem. An important component of the occupational health problem is the issue of information: its collection, dissemination, and interpretation for use in decisions. The purpose of this chapter is to deal analytically with those informational issues, on the assumption that they may have significant implications for the future of all kinds of employer-employee communications about health.

Occupational Health: Defining the Problem

Worksite health hazards can be classified in various ways, but Ashford's scheme is as useful as any. He enumerates four categories of occupational exposure:

physical—noise, heat, vibration, and radiation

chemical—dusts, poisonous fumes and gases, toxic metals and chemicals, and carcinogens

biological—bacteria, fungi and insects

stress—including that caused by physical, chemical, and ergonomic factors, and psychological factors such as disciplinary pressure on the job.[1]

Most attention is currently being directed at physical and chemical hazards, Ashford says, "in part because these hazards or their effects are most easily detected or measured by the senses or by analytical instrumentation."[2]

Though not so easily detected, carcinogens (cancer-causing agents) doubtless occasion the greatest alarm of all because of their especially damaging effects with little or no advance notice. The unique problem of occupational cancer was explored by a special committee of the National Academy of Sciences,[3] which presented the eight concepts quoted in the box as the foundation for a broad understanding of the problem.

Substances with possible mutagenic (causing biological mutation) or teratogenic (causing fetal deformities) properties or other effects on human fertility also elicit grave concern on three levels: first, because birth defects are particularly agonizing; second, because interference with fertility could foreshadow a substance's carcinogenic potential. For example, on recently learning that working with the pesticide DBCP was the probable cause of his sterility, an Occidental Chemical Company employee reportedly said: "I'm only worried about one thing. If DBCP can cause sterility, then just what else can it cause?"[4]

Third, and perhaps most important, is the spectre of widespread genetic alteration caused by exposures to chemicals or radiation: "Surely one of the

UNDERSTANDING OCCUPATIONAL CANCER
EIGHT ESSENTIAL CONCEPTS

Many carcinogenic substances can be absorbed by man without any warning signal such as coughing, burning, or nausea.

If permanent damage is done to a cell by a carcinogenic agent, the defect is passed on to daughter cells in the process of multiplication. The effects of repeated exposure can, therefore, be additive. Moreover, some agents, such as asbestos, are not readily eliminated from the body, so their concentrations increase with repeated exposure.

There is usually a latent period from five to thirty or more years between the first absorption of the carcinogen and the appearance of any sign of disease.

Although there is still some debate within scientific circles, for all practical purposes there is no dose of a carcinogen below which one can say that there is absolutely no risk of its causing cancer. Nevertheless, decreasing the exposure decreases the risk, and increasing it increases the risk.

The hazard of a carcinogen is, in some instances, multiplied if it is absorbed in conjunction with other substances, such as cigarette smoke.

Some carcinogens can be inadvertently transferred from the workplace to the home in significant quantities.

An indication that a substance may produce cancer in man is frequently found in experiments on laboratory animals and cells. When an agent is demonstrated, in controlled experiments, to produce cancer in animals, that agent should be regarded as possibly carcinogenic in man.

In some instances, benign tumors develop into cancer; and in many instances agents that produce benign tumors increase the risk of cancer.

SOURCE: Division of Medical Sciences, Assembly of Life Sciences, National Research Council, Committee on Public Information in the Prevention of Occupational Cancer: *Informing Workers and Employers About Occupational Cancer.* Washington, D.C.: National Academy of Sciences, 1977, pp. 7–8.

greatest responsibilities of our generation," observed an HEW-appointed committee on pesticides and environmental health, "is our temporary custody of the genetic heritage received from our ancestors."[5] A committee of the American College of Obstetricians and Gynecologists (ACOG), with funding from the National Institute of Occupational Safety and Health, recently completed a project to develop guidelines on pregnancy and work for use by practicing physicians. The guidelines are available from ACOG,[6] and the committee's deliberations have been described in published accounts by its chairman, Leon J. Warshaw, M.D. vice president and corporate medical director of The Equitable Life Assurance Society of the United States.[7]

Apart from the important but reasonably straightforward clinical concerns about managing the pregnancy of a working woman, and the rather remote considerations of greviously altered gene pools, a welter of emotionally charged issues of rights in conflict arise from the possible effects on fertility and the fetus of workplace exposures. Lead is the substance now most in the news in this connection. Unions and feminist groups have questioned General Motors' right to exclude women workers of childbearing age from holding jobs in battery plants where they might be exposed to airborne lead. A Canadian mother of four underwent surgical sterilization in order to secure her GM job, and later charged the corporation with sex discrimination. According to a *Wall Street Journal* account, Dr. H.C. Scharnweber, a corporate medical director of Dow Chemical Company, "sees employers caught in a legal crossfire. If they permit exposure to occupational dangers, they face lawsuits 'on behalf of every unsuccessful pregnancy.' If they bar women workers from hazardous jobs, they face sex discrimination charges by workers or their unions."[8]

This no-win situation is faintly evocative of the legal gauntlet it was argued employers will have to run should they become involved in influencing employees' choices of physicians in the community. The employer may be reluctant to pass along negative opinions of an individual provider for fear of opening himself to libel suits. Neither may he want to endorse an individual source of care because if the course of the medical treatment should go wrong, he might be subject to a malpractice suit. In this situation, as in the occupational health domain, the dilemmas are real and might seem best avoided in the name of prudence and safe employee relations. But the press of events and of changing expectations seem likely to make it impossible for at least some industries in some geographical areas to avoid these confrontations indefinitely.

In addition to the special problem of occupationally related cancer, some nonmalignant occupational health conditions are of serious concern, for example, lung diseases such as asbestosis, silicosis, coalworkers' pneumoconiosis, and byssinosis, skin diseases, and chemical burns, and a wide variety of physical and psychological stresses. From the perspective of informing employees, however, the most worrisome occupational diseases are those, like cancer, that are insidious and ambiguous in onset, leaving workers largely unaware of the dangers. The exact etiology of these diseases is complex; they usually have multiple causes, long latency periods, and varying effects on individuals exposed. Information is sparse on what constitutes a dangerous chronic exposure to low levels of these agents and on how they may interact

OCCUPATIONAL HEALTH HAZARDS
ESTIMATING THE EXTENT OF THE PROBLEM

Editor's Note: The data here are preliminary estimates based on imperfect information. NIOSH carefully qualifies them in its report, which should be consulted before general conclusions are drawn.

Workers (Host)

Of 84 million[1] American workers, NIOSH estimates approximately

880,000 (1%) "face full or part-time exposure to an OSHA-regulated carcinogen."[1]

21 million (25%) "currently may be exposed full-time or part-time to hazardous substances."[1]

40–50 million (23% of the general population) "may have had exposure to one or more . . . hazardous substances during their working lifetimes."[1]

25.2 million (30%) work in "small-workplaces, employing 25 or fewer people."[2]

Hazardous Materials (Agent)

63,000 chemicals are thought to be in common use.

Over 25,000 different chmicals were listed in 1976 in the Annual Registry of Toxic Effects of Chemical Substances.[1]

Nearly 2,000 are suspected carcinogens.[1]

400 toxic substances are regulated by OSHA via "consensus standards" promulgated when the Act was passed. These consist only of environmental limits.[1]

with other exposures, within the worksite and beyond, to produce multiplying and synergistic combinations.

How prevalent these diseases and their causative agents are and how large the population at risk remain largely conjectural. Friedland's paper, in part II, discusses available statistics and their limitations. For convenience, the data can be conceptualized within the traditional public health paradigm of host, agent, environment, as in the box.

The figures in the box are very rough estimates which just begin to flesh out the dimensions of the occupational health problem. The importance of the problem transcends these estimates of direct exposure into the broader social

Over 60 criteria documents recommending comprehensive standards have been transmitted from NIOSH to OSHA but have not been acted on. At least 9 of these deal with suspected carcinogens.

17 toxic substances are now regulated by OSHA through comprehensive permanent standards.

Work Sites (Environment)

5 million work sites come under OSHA's jurisdiction[2] (i.e., are U.S. employers engaged in business affecting interstate commerce)

4 million are "small," (i.e., 24 or fewer employees).

Industrial hygiene services are available in an estimated:[1]

2% workplaces with 8–249 employees
15% workplaces with 250–500 employees
42% workplaces with 500+ employees

Estimated exposures of full-time workers:[1]

Toxic Substances	Estimated Workers Exposed	With No Protection
asbestos	83,494	90%
benzene	48,484	55%
cutting oil	144,535	75%
carcinogens (OSHA-regulated)	880,000	NA

[1]National Institute for Occupational Safety and Health: "The Right to Know: Policy Issues Arising from Exposures to Hazardous Chemical and Physical Agents in the Workplace," Rockville, Md.: National Institute of Occupational Safety and Health, July 1977.

[2]Holsendolph, Ernest: "Washington and Business: Job Safety Aid for Small Concerns," New York Times (August 25, 1977): 51.

problems of environmental protection and consumer product safety in which occupational health is embedded. The workplace, where exposures tend to higher concentrations, greater frequency, and more extended periods, can serve as an early warning system for incipient troubles in the outside environment. Conversely, the workplace affords greater control over exposures than is normally possible outside. Together, these conditions militate for vigorous pursuit of preventive efforts in the workplace, for the sake of the affected workers, irrespective of their numbers, and for the sake of society more generally. A National Institutes of Health and American College of Preventive Medicine task force recently reported on occupational health as part of a comprehensive series of reports entitled, *Preventive Medicine U.S.A.* The first step toward better prevention, according to that group, is to generate fuller information and a sounder base of knowledge:

> The sequence of solving an occupational health problem is conceptually simple; that is, health effects are ascertained along with measurements of exposure. If specific conditions or exposures relate to excess disease or injury then these conditions or exposures are reduced or eliminated to reduce or eliminate the disease or injury. There are many examples of how this has been done. There are even more examples of failure to apply this approach. . . . One of our biggest deficiencies is lack of basic information on connections between occupational exposures and disease.[9]

Scientific Evidence and Weak Links in the Chain of Causality

How these causal connections are traced—from initial suspicion to discovery of clusters of evidence, to validation of an association, and then to overall assessment of risk—has been elaborated in many different contexts. A recent effort that is readable, relevant to occupational health, and well-documented is a book entitled, *Of Acceptable Risk: Science and the Determination of Safety*, by William W. Lowrance.[10] From a different perspective, the President's Scientific Advisory Committee report, *Chemicals and Health*, emphasizes, as does Lowrance, the need for greater appreciation of the "dynamic nature of science and the changing character of scientific understanding . . . the probabilistic rather than clear-cut or definitive character of scientific judgments."[11]

Caveats such as these are offered to discourage unwarranted generalization from limited scientific findings, elevating them to rigid dogma. The Delaney Amendment to the Food and Drug Act is frequently cited in evidence that this is not an idle fear. The Delaney clause, according to the President's Advisory Committee, invites "overliteral interpretations," which are "a refuge in the face of ignorance."[12] Introduced by Congressman Delaney in 1958, the controversial law stipulates that "no [food] additive shall be deemed to be safe if it is found . . . after tests which are appropriate for the evaluation of the safety of food additives, to induce cancer in animal or man."[13] Subsequent regulations extended the principle to feed for promoting animal growth and to food colorings The assumptions behind the clause and the source of the controversy are the twin notions that the only tolerable exposure level to a carcinogen is zero, and that animal tests are sufficient to "prove" carcinogenicity.

To some extent, the debate over what constitutes definitive evidence of carcinogenicity bears testimony to important progress in scientific technique and technical knowledge that has been achieved in recent years. This has brought substantial improvement in the capacity to detect small traces of elements in the environment and subtle effects on humans. In parallel with increased sophistication in epidemiological research, this progress has kindled new awareness of dangers that only recently would have been unimaginable.[14] Still, the pieces of the research puzzle are scattered and are being gathered slowly, as data are gradually accumulated through epidemiological studies of populations, supplemented by laboratory experimentation on animal, bacterial, and cell culture systems, each somewhat limited in its predictive power for man or for the particular circumstances of the exposures being questioned.

Notwithstanding progressive refinements in methodology, scientific resources may seem limited in the face of an occupational health problem that some characterize as boundless and growing:

> We can never create enough data fast enough to solve the expanding problem. We are bathed in a sea of chemicals, and the National Cancer Institute cancer map, the accidentally discovered evidence from various industries, and the cancer mortality of both United States and foreign chemists all suggest that we are in deep trouble. The cancer problems we are seeing today are probably from exposures fifteen or twenty years ago. Do you realize what that means for industrial cancer over the next few decades during which we will experience cancer whose origin is traceable to the expanding use of chemicals which has increased fourfold every decade since 1945?
>
> Nicholas A. Ashford

> It's almost a carcinogen-of-the-week phenomenon we're experiencing nowadays.
>
> Rick J. Carlson

These comments represent one extreme view. At the other pole, the case can be made that the considerable attention now being paid the problem of environmentally provoked cancer will probably yield the improved knowledge and abatement technology needed to substantially mitigate future exposures and gradually bring the problem under some measure of control. In hopes of marshaling available scientific resources as efficiently as possible, efforts are now being made to establish firm grounding for rational research priorities. The effort derives in part from a recognition that "detailed and systematic knowledge of health effects from environmental chemical agents lags far behind the levels of quantification and reliability accessible to contemporary science."[15]

Implicitly accepting this assumption, for example, the *Preventive Medicine, U.S.A.* task force on environmental health proposed a multidisciplinary research effort targeted to suspicious and widespread agents where the potential research payoff should be high. The targets would be identified through a combination of traditional research approaches, in concert with analysis of chemical composition and toxicological characteristics of agents and of economic factors such as prevalence in the workplace, contribution to the economy, and predicted future markets. In arguing the merits of such an approach, the task force observed:

> On the basis of economic projections, polyvinyl chloride should have been easily seen as a plastic of rising production and great commercial importance. Rising production usually means more exposed workers and thus higher potential value to screening. There are materials being introduced today which are in all likelihood the polyvinyl chlorides of tomorrow.[16]

An effort to set research priorities for engineering controls[17] was recently inaugurated by NIOSH with a survey it commissioned to pinpoint hazardous industries in terms of exposures to carcinogens. Undertaken by the Research Triangle Institute, the study reportedly ranked eighty-six industrial chemicals by their apparent carcinogenic potency and combined these ratings with data on the numbers of workers in different industries exposed and the length of exposures. Previous research had tended to consider the volume of the carcinogens in the workplace, divorced from aggregate exposure levels. An interesting difference in the results of this new approach was a safer profile of the chemical industry—not listed there among the eight most hazardous—then is commonly reached by methods taking account of the extremely large volumes of dangerous chemicals commonly used in that industry's production processes, but not of the fact that often relatively few workers handle them directly.[18]

Seeking to establish regulatory priorities in a milieu of scientific uncertainty, the Occupational Safety and Health Administration (OSHA), in October 1977, proposed new rules for regulating industrial carcinogens. In its six-year history, OSHA has set final standards for only 17 of perhaps 1,500 to 2,000 carcinogens believed now in industrial use in the United States. The proposal would expedite the standard-setting process, but, like most of OSHA's activities, it is now enveloped in controversy.

The new policy would replace OSHA's current substance-by-substance rulemaking approach with a standardized series of regulatory steps for carcinogens in four categories. Categorization in each of the first three would depend principally on the strength of the scientific evidence suggesting carcinogenicity; the fourth would subsume all cancer-causing substances not found in United States workplaces.

The specifics of the proposal and the details of OSHA's difficulties are beyond the scope of this volume. But it seems clear that OSHA's search for more rational and efficient ways to allocate its limited resources will continue and escalate over the next several years. From the standpoint of communicating to employees about occupational health hazards, OSHA's proposal is relevant because the essential principle—that dangerous materials should be treated differentially, depending on the strength of the scientific evidence indicting them—can be usefully applied to the problem of when and how best to warn workers of hazards they may be confronting.

Dissemination of Information: Why, When, Who, and How

No question can remain at this point of the importance of warning workers when conditions of their employment jeopardize their health. Recognizing this, and acknowledging the regrettable—sometimes tragic and unconscionable—episodes in the past in which workers may have been unwittingly misled, even deliberately deceived, about work-related dangers to their health, one still finds dilemmas and honest disagreement among people of good will. The real controversy, now, revolves around the definition of evidence considered convincing enough to pass on to workers and to require modifications in the workplace. Scientific standards of truth are one thing, workers' informational needs, another:

> The prime problem is this: at what stage of scientific certainty does one transmit the information to the worker? As scientists, we are trained to adhere to very rigorous standards of causality. On the other hand, the law is willing to accept indications of causality on what is called "the frontiers of science." The very difficult question then becomes, what degree of certitude must we have before there exists this duty to inform? And my feeling is that all the information should be transmitted, with the degrees of disagreement spelled out clearly, and along with it any interpretation that exists.
> Nicholas A. Ashford

Ashford's prescription here is basically the same as that advanced by Annas and others in relation to physician advertising: let the information out with all its imperfections showing, let "the experts" comment freely, and let the people who are most directly affected interpret it finally for themselves. But, as in the case of physician advertising, conflicting rights, economic interests, and views of reality complicate the situation. There are legal obligations to inform workers, as Blum and Friedland argue independently in part II, and legal disincentives as well:

> Certainly, it would have to be acknowledged by management, I would think, that they are not concerned about one or two employees out of a thousand hopping to some other employer when news of a health hazard breaks. On the other hand, they probably are worried, with some considerable justification, about legal liability as well as repercussions at the union level and, over the longer haul, the danger that people generally may begin to question the social utility of the products they are making. Those are probably legitimate worries.
> Rick J. Carlson

Leaving legal liability aside, major economic consequences flow from the decision to inform a group of workers, as clearly indicated by the recent NIOSH estimates summarized in the box. If informing the workers were simply a matter of opening a floodgate and loosing dammed up information, the issues would be far simpler and the stakes not nearly as high.

Also arguing for caution is a feeling that premature or inappropriate notification of workers could be counterproductive of health protection by contributing to unnecessary fear, general confusion, or, over time, a sense of either complacency or futility from information overload.

For these and other reasons, it is not enough simply to assert that the worker ought always to be told everything in relation to his health. A more sophisticated approach is necessary, and the OSHA model for the new cancer regulations provides a useful beginning framework. In deciding what to tell workers and how, there are at least three different levels of hazard, each with its own set of imperatives and of demands.

INFORMING WORKERS EXPOSED TO HEALTH HAZARDS: TOTAL COST ESTIMATES FOR DIFFERENT GROUPS OF WORKERS*

	Workers in NIOSH Epidemiological Studies (in 000)	Workers Currently Exposed to OSHA-Regulated Carcinogens Full-time (in 000)	Workers Currently Exposed to OSHA-Regulated Carcinogens Full-time or Part-time (in 000)	Workers Currently Exposed to OSHA-Regulated Substances Full-time (in 000)	Workers Currently Exposed to OSHA-Regulated Substances Full-time or Part-time (in 000)
Number of Workers**	101	44	880	1,050	21,000
Obtain Addresses	$ 40	$ 18	$ 352	$ 420	$ 8,400
Compose Letters	3	3	3	6	6
Print & Mail	152	66	1,320	1,575	31,500
Hotline	114	50	990	1,181	23,625
Conferences	200	200	200	375	375
Surveillance	415,769	423,280	8,465,600	2,580,500	54,193,000
TOTAL	$416,278	$423,617	$8,468,465	$2,584,057	$54,256,906
Approximate years	17	37	37	37	37
Approximate Annual Cost	$ 24,000	$ 11,000	$ 229,000	$ 70,000	$ 1,466,000

*Groupings used here are not mutually exclusive and should not be summed.
**Cost of locating names of all workers included in NIOSH studies not included.
SOURCE: National Institute for Occupational Safety and Health, Center for Disease Control, U.S. Department of Health, Education, and Welfare: *The Right to Know; Practical Problems and Policy Issues Arising from Exposures to Hazardous Chemical and Physical Agents in the Workplace*, July 1977, table 5, page 31.

Editor's Note: The NIOSH report spells out the assumptions and caveats underlying these rough estimates and should be consulted by anyone wishing to make use of the figures.

Levels of Hazard and Degrees of Urgency

On the first level is the clear and present danger, the highest priority problem in the classification scheme. The facts are known, the interpretation is accepted, and the imperative both to inform affected workers and to modify the workplace as rapidly and fully as possible is absolutely unequivocal. Asbestos is a good example—indeed, the seventeen carcinogens for which OSHA has set final standards would all come under this first rubric. Ethical imperatives, practical considerations, and the law establish the duty to inform workers exposed to these hazards. Informing the worker is one step in the process of making the workplace safe because it enables him to participate in his own protection. But, as the NIOSH estimates assume, informing the workers is only one of several necessary steps in the case of very hazardous materials. The employer is also obliged to provide counseling and follow-up services, including systematic medical surveillance, and to institute controls to eliminate dangerous levels of exposure. In fact, these long-term obligations after the message has been communicated constitute the bulk of the expense deriving from the obligation to inform workers.

The second-level problem is where shades of grey begin to appear. There is some evidence of danger at this level, but still some ambiguity:

> I noticed in your paper, Dr. Karrh, a significant hedge point. You talked about "firm evidence for carcinogenicity," and really, I think you failed to note that there are pivotal points and areas of disagreement here.
>
> Arthur E. Gass

> I'm not convinced that a company is being that helpful in communicating to the employee information that is not fully understood. Take the Ames test. The results vary with the different laboratories running the tests, and the messages we're getting are pretty mixed. We can communicate all that to the employee, but if we do, the chances are he'll come back to us and say, "Okay, doc, you've given me this information, but now tell me what it means, as far as my job, my health, my kids, my wife, and everything. What does it really mean?" What do you tell that worker?
>
> Bruce W. Karrh

The zone of uncertainty is wide, as suggested by estimates that OSHA's new cancer regulations will cover perhaps as many as 300 different substances, instead of the 17 now regulated, and the NIOSH estimate that there may be more than 2,000 carcinogens in the American workplace. The magnitude of the uncertainty seems to argue forcefully for informing workers as fully as possible and enlisting them as partners in dealing with a major problem.

The third-level problem, finally, is nearly pure ambiguity—speculation or foreboding based on very thin empirical evidence. Here the first imperative is to improve the information base, although here, too, a good case can be made for letting the worker share the concern:

> Let's take a specific example, vinyl bromide, a first cousin, chemi-
> cally, of vinyl chloride, which is a demonstrated carcinogen, regu-
> lated by OSHA. Vinyl bromide, so far, has escaped indictment. I
> don't know if it's a carcinogen or not. But, if I were working in a
> vinyl bromide plant, I'd surely want to know that there are grounds
> for suspicion. I'd want to be pretty careful in the way I handled that
> chemical.
>
> Nicholas A. Ashford

Having granted the importance of information at each of the various levels,
serious problems remain about how to communicate it:

> Most people I talk with in industry are now moving quite far in the
> direction of trying to inform their employees totally. Most are
> trying to make sure employees know what health hazards they are
> associated with to the extent of industry's knowledge or ability to
> inform the employees at the time. But it's not an easy task. There
> are several specific questions that are difficult to answer: Whom do
> you tell—all employees, including those no longer being exposed,
> or only those now being exposed? What about former employees
> with whom you no longer have formal contact nor adequate com-
> munication mechanisms? How do you find them? What about
> pensioners? And then how do you tell them, and what, exactly, do
> you tell them? There are no simple answers to these questions.
>
> Bruce W. Karrh

Communciation Arenas and Issues of Implementation

For the sake of analysis, Karrh's questions and ancillary issues can be
broken down into four communication arenas, each with its own set of policy
issues and mechanical or technical communication questions. The emphasis of
this volume is on the issues rather than on the techniques of disseminating
information. For additional information on specific techniques, Friedland, in
part II, cites a number of useful sources, among which the NIOSH report[19] and
some segments of the proceedings of the conference convened by the Committee on Public Information in the Prevention of Occupational Cancer[20] may be
particularly useful.

Within the Firm

As Karrh suggests, the thorniest questions for internal communication
are: who is to do the informing, who is to be informed, and what is to be the
substantive message? The kinds of questions that arise are typified by this
exchange:

> Dr. Karrh, I have great respect for your system and your company
> and your medical care. It ranks, clearly, with Exxon, Dow, and
> other good companies we know about. But I am a little appalled to

hear you say that you have a foreman deliver a message like, "Hey, you've been exposed to very toxic levels of a carcinogen."

Arthur E. Gass

We think this is the best way for us to do it. At DuPont, the employee's contact with management, no matter what the issue, is with the supervisor. For an occupational health communication, the supervisor remains the first point of contact, and after that the employee can go to the medical department, the industrial hygien-ist, or the toxicologist for clarification. We think this is the best way to communicate in our company. The important thing isn't how it is done, but rather that it gets the information across as effectively and sensitively as possible.

Bruce M. Karrh

The fact that DuPont and similarly large corporations have well-estab-lished mechanisms for communicating with employees sets them apart from small plants and firms. The Committee on Public Information in the Prevention of Occupational Cancer explored the problem of how to inform the nonunion and small plant worker, and found this to be the knottiest problem of all because effective mechanisms and channels for communication are lacking and resources are thin.[21] More than 50 million of the nation's 70 million workers do not belong to a union and the bulk of nonunion employees work in small plants and shops.[22]

Other intrafirm issues include the counseling and medical follow-up responsibilities that have already been alluded to in connection with the NIOSH estimates of the costs of informing workers and the need for developing effective industrial hygiene monitoring and controls. As Friedland points out in part II, informed workers can contribute significantly to workplace monitor-ing and to developing practicable controls.

Across Firms or Industries

There is another set of issues applying to communication among firms. These are related to trade secrecy, generic labeling, and sharing of proprietary information that may have important ramifications for the health of large numbers of workers. These problems surfaced publicly when NIOSH was conducting its National Occupational Hazard Survey, begun in 1972 and only recently completed. NIOSH was stymied repeatedly by the inability to deter-mine the chemical composition of substances widely used in industrial pro-duction. John Finklea, then director of NIOSH, told a congressional oversight committee of the agency's frustrations:

A major problem in completing the study ... is that companies surveyed often were not aware of the chemical composition of the substances used in their plant. Over 70 percent of the exposures identified were recorded as trade name products for which the chemical composition was not known to the company. Approximately one-third of the products we surveyed were designated as trade secrets. ... We estimate that more than seven million workers in the United States are exposed to trade name products containing an OSHA regulated toxic substance. Even more disturbing, our survey indicates that there may be more than 300,000 workers exposed to trade name products containing one of the sixteen carcinogens regulated by OSHA [at the time of the testimony]. . . . In these cases, neither the employer nor the employee may have been aware of the ingredients of these products.[23]

Subsequent to Finklea's testimony, Eula Bingham, assistant secretary of labor for occupational safety and health, reported to the same committee the results of legal analysis which concluded that "OSHA has the legal authority . . . to require manufacturers, formulators, and sellers of industrial products to disclose to the purchasers of these products, through labels or data sheets, the presence of toxic substances.[24] The Toxic Substances Control Act of 1976, when its implementation mechanisms are fully in place, will provide additional legal authority, but perhaps not the administrative coordination necessary to accomplish this task of information dissemination. In any case, the problem remains for the present and obviously constrains many employers in fulfilling an obligation to warn employees of hazards.

Another interfirm concern is the related question of whether to share information on production processes and engineering controls when hazardous materials are involved. The demands of a competitive market militate against such purely altruistic gestures, but in a perfect world, one would hope that they might be made nevertheless:

> When I try to be objective, I can see why a corporation might hestiate to publicize innovations in engineering controls and give up the profit edge it might otherwise enjoy. On the other hand, wouldn't it be a humane contribution to public health to pass these engineering controls around the industry, so that other workers would not have to suffer high-risk exposures?
>
> Arthur E. Gass

Between Industry and Government

It is firm-to-government communication and vice versa that is clearly the most contentious. Regulation, in many cases, creates an adversary relationship; conflict is to be expected, perhaps even to be desired. Also, not surprisingly, discord over rights and responsibilities often spills over from other arenas into this one. The legal contretemps over confidentiality of workers' health records, alluded to in chapter 1, illustrates the point.

In May 1976, NIOSH began a health survey of a DuPont Company plant in Belle, West Virginia. The employee who requested the survey was concerned that cancer seemed unusually widespread among his fellow workers. After initial explorations, NIOSH approached DuPont for medical records and work histories of past and present employees at the Belle plant, and the company wrote to some 3,000 such employees soliciting their consent to the release of the records. When 631 respondents refused consent, DuPont denied NIOSH access to their records. NIOSH issued an administrative subpoena for the records, and DuPont went to court on February 8, 1977, for a declaratory judgment asking the courts to resolve the conflict between the corporation's legal duty to comply with NIOSH's subpoena and its responsibility to protect its employees' privacy. The court rendered a judgment in December 1977 which upheld NIOSH's right of access to the disputed records but stipulated specific measures to insulate them from third parties.

Fundamentally at issue in the case is the scope of the government's authority under OSHAct to extract medical records from industry. DuPont officials said that they had offered to release the information in a format that would have permitted statistical analysis without identifying individuals. But the government researchers wanted full control over their investigation.[25] The case could set an important precedent; indeed, in October 1977, a General Motors plant in Dayton, Ohio, went to court with an analogous petition. Also at issue are broader questions of informed consent for human subjects research and the employer's role in assuring the confidentiality of the employee's health records.

Confidentiality of health records has received intense scrutiny especially since the enactment of the Federal Privacy Act of 1974. A Privacy Protection Commission, created by the act, produced a comprehensive report[26] in which medical records figured prominently because, the chairman said, "of all record-keeping relationships, medical records are the most intrusive."[27] The National Bureau of Standards subsequently contracted with a group at Columbia University to conduct a pilot study of one aspect of the general dilemma of protecting citizens' rights in a computerized age. That group chose to examine health records, believing them critically important because of increased elaboration and automation already occurring in programs like the professional standards review organizations and likely to accelerate as the nation moves toward some form of national financing system for health services. Also, the report said, "health is a universal experience. Since the use of health care data affects everyone's rights, benefits, and opportunities in the larger society, this presents all the subtle and difficult problems of how to regulate secondary uses of personal information."[27]

The Privacy Commission was dissolved with the publication of its report, so to supplement its efforts, with specific reference to health records, the American Psychiatric Association and other private groups created a National Commission on Confidentiality of Health Records, located in Washington, D.C. That commission sponsored a conference in October 1977 at which the general matter of employee health records, and specifically the DuPont-NIOSH face-off, "pervaded the discussions."[29] According to published accounts, the sense of the meeting was that research needs may at times outweigh concerns for privacy and informed consent. Union participants were reportedly most militant in their espousal of this view, and they asserted that the real issue is not simply confidentiality and personal privacy but the possibility that aggressive research might uncover evidence that could make it necessary for industry to spend a lot of money abating newly defined health hazards.

Between Industry and the Medical System

From industry to the outside medical system and back, communication is widely believed to be badly in need of improvement:

The channels of communication between the occupational physician and the rest of the medical profession for transmission of information about the health hazards of the workplace ... [are] a problem because an uncertain proportion of occupational physicians are restricted from such communication by their employers for reasons of liability for damages, unfavorable publicity, potential requirements for plant redesign, production delays, and so forth. They are also a problem because at least a portion of these potential communications have major significance to the total medical community.[30]

Some lay the problem principally at the doorstep of industry, more specifically, of occupational medicine.

A great deal of effort has to be expended in establishing more firmly the credibility and ethical standards of occupational medicine. All too often we find that the private physician does not fully trust the findings of tests performed by the corporate medical department and repeats them on the outside. This is one symptom—a costly one—of a larger problem. Too many people feel that the occupational medical establishment withholds information and may even manipulate it.

Saul M. Kilstein

Others assert that deficiencies exist on both sides. Arthur Gass made that point in the context of the labeling problem already discussed:

Products ought to be labeled properly with generic or Geneva names so that workers can take this information to their private physicians when the doctor says, "Hey, what are you being exposed to on your job?" Now that, of course, is making a big assumption—that the private physician knows enough about toxicology to ask the question. A recent survey we performed showed that only 5 or 6 of the nation's 120 or so medical schools require toxicology training. The others may give an hour or two in a pharmacology course, or invite in a guest lecturer or two, but it's not an obligatory course. And it's a difficult subject, so the students don't tend to elect it unless they have to.

The first volume in this series sketched the evolution of occupational medicine and pointed to evidence of small chinks in the massive wall that has traditionally separated the occupational physician's domain from the general medical system. The specialty's newly developed code of ethics, quoted fully in that volume, takes a long first step toward a more tenable position, and it seems a safe prediction that the rapidly unfolding occupational health problems, together with escalating health care costs, will continue to inspire a healthy reexamination of the role of the occupational physician, in search of more efficient and more effective relationships with the mainstream medical system.

Application of Information: The Bottom Line

Behind the scientific endeavor to improve the knowledge base, and the legal and ethical imperatives pressing for dissemination of available information, the fundamental purpose—the "bottom line"—is to stimulate preventive action. A basic assumption is that the information has utility, that it will facilitate a better decision, whether by the individual worker, the employer, society, or some combination. The decision process often requires weighing of a subtle blend of objective evidence, individual preferences, and a very rough estimate of a possibly wide margin for error.

Personal Decisions

In occupational health as in medical care, market imperfections point to the need for better information. A perfectly efficient labor market would reveal explicitly the hazards encountered on a given job and would offer salary premiums in proportion to the amount of risk a worker willingly and knowingly assumes, up to the level where the firm would choose to invest in abating the risks as a financially preferable alternative to augmenting salaries and providing full compensation.[31] As discussed in the first volume of this series, workers' compensation laws operate on this principle. They seek to internalize the costs of occupational accidents and illness so that the firm will have an incentive to invest in safety precautions. Only in relation to occupational accidents, where consequences are visible and immediate, have they succeeded in this, and there only to a degree.

With regard to occupational health, the theoretical formulation of an efficient labor market runs into several practical problems. First, it compares money with health and life and, therefore, arouses suspicion and discomfort. These objections, however, can be partially countered with the observation that cost-benefit analyses, in real life as in economic theory, often demand a willingness to bridge a logical gap. Another practical problem, less easily handled, is the shortage of useful information with which to deliberate about relative costs and benefits of the available options.

An illustration emerges from the debate over whether and when personal protective devices (such as respirators or ear plugs) are appropriate in lieu of engineering controls (such as architectural modifications to the facility) or administrative controls (alterations in shifts, breaks from specific tasks, and other changes in work practices). Unions tend to oppose personal protection approaches on principle, arguing that the firm ought to absorb the costs of making the workplace safe, rather than passing the burden along to the worker in the form of discomfort or inconvenience on the job. Moreover, uncomfortable personal protective devices are not always used consistently and are therefore less effective. On the other hand, engineering controls and, to a lesser extent, administrative controls, often cost more. Management may feel that the cost differential is excessive and that the added expense would jeopardize the overall financial security of the firm. But analytical tools are lacking to trace its precise impact on workers as wage earners, taxpayers, consumers, and owners of pension funds. Consequently, the case is often left to be argued largely on ideological or emotional grounds.

The trade-offs that are made are often tacit and remote: for each unmeasurable increment of protection against an unknowable risk, there are the costs of the controls and their potential consequences for the firm's profits, wages, and competitive position in the market, as well as more globally for employment. For the inconvenience and discomfort of personal protective devices, the

WHY INFORM? THE USES OF INFORMATION

Nicholas A. Ashford: I do not believe that workers, or anyone else, can relate to the low probability of chronic risk situations. This is where I disagree with the writings of Robert Smith.[41] Though I believe firmly in transmitting the information, I think it has very minimal effect on personal behavior. The main reasons for requiring its transmission are, first, to help in establishing legal liability, which does serve as a kind of deterrent, and, second, to arouse public opinion to the severity of the problem.

Robert S. Smith: I tend to agree with Nick Ashford that full information is absolutely useful and essential for the social welfare. Where we differ, I think, is that I would be quite willing to accept the worker's judgment, as evidenced by his behavior. Nick seems to argue that no one should be allowed to work in a vinyl bromide plant, because this may be a dangerous substance, and anyone electing to work with it would have to be deemed irrational no matter what the incentives. I believe that the purpose of informing workers of the risks is to allow them to make decisions that they feel are in their own self-interest, rather than defining for them what we consider rational behavior on their part.

Morris E. Chafetz: When I hear the statement, "Why inform people, they don't change," I bridle because I consider this the fundamental impediment to social progress: the self-fulfilling prophesy. I guarantee you that if you set up a system to bring about change with the idea that people won't, they will live up to your expectations. We provide information, and people don't change, and we never think to ask, "Why should they?" That's paternalism that smacks of a putdown, and it's no wonder that people don't respond.

aggregate costs may be lower, but so may the benefits. Administrative controls may cut into productivity by reducing the efficiency in work practices. What they lose in flexibility and freedom to choose work assignments, workers may or may not recover some day in longevity and health, and they are understandably chary of medical screening programs, fearing transfer to a lower paying and less desirable job.

Many occupational health hazards pose invisible and low-probability risks over a long time horizon. Their deferred onset raises serious questions about the individual's ability to give them appropriate credence. How to

---

Dr. Ashford: It comes down to whether you believe people can make rational decisions for themselves under these circumstances. There is a whole body of literature on risk analysis dealing with people who live near earthquake faults and so forth, and it demonstrates quite convincingly that people have difficulty relating to long-term low-probability risk. We just have to agree or disagree on whether people can in fact be rational on this. But, even if I were for the moment to grant a rational response to a health risk, we then come down to the question of distributional wealth. If someone who doesn't have enough bread to eat is faced with a small risk on his job, he is likely to say, "Look, the cancer risk is a long way off. Today I need the bread." That worker is making the only decision that is before him. He has one viable alternative. And if you think that's O.K., then you think what Smith says is O.K. But that means you don't care about the fact that the people who sell their health and the people who buy that health come from different social strata.

Bruce W. Karrh: Dr. Ashford is arguing that the person reaping the benefit is not the one taking the risk. I disagree. Employees benefit from the compensations of their jobs, whatever those jobs may be. Sure, there are complex issues here, but we have to begin with the premise that the job has value for the worker.

Rick J. Carlson: I know how I respond to a health risk, even if the probability is low. Tris is a good example, though not an occupational one. You've got consumers and a chemical, but the principles are not all that different. I, for one, would have given a lot to have learned about Tris earlier than I did. If I had known that my two kids were being exposed to a statistically very small cancer risk, I would have burned those pajamas a lot sooner than I did. A lot of people would have acted on that information if they had had it, and they didn't get it, for a variety of reasons, until very late in the game.

proceed from this observation is controversial, as the quotations in the box demonstrate. The position Ashford takes there is carried even farther by spokesmen for organized labor, like Anthony Mazzocchi of the Oil, Chemical and Atomic Workers' Union. He was recently reported in the *New York Times* to have said that "balancing the number of lives a regulation might save against the money it would cost an industry [is] 'calculated murder.'"[32] The article continues, "many economists and some government officials, however, contend that, in an age when there are several thousand suspected carcinogens, such calculations are essential."[33] Refusing to face the choices squarely simply prevents them from being made explicitly.

Painful though they are to make, estimates of the amount of expenditure different regulations exact in pursuit of a statistically measured saving of life are useful for comparing various government requirements. Interventions can then be designed with the greatest potential impact per dollar spent. No one wants to place a value on a human life but economists assert that the notion of a "statistical life" is an abstraction or an analytical tool that helps sharpen the precision of difficult decisions.[34]

Ashford, as quoted in the box, argues that even informed workers may lack wide enough discretion to choose the course of action best for their health. This echoes sentiments voiced by John Finklea, former director of NIOSH, who spoke in congressional testimony of "gaps" in the compensation system:

> If a worker shows some impairment of function but . . . no disease, [he] may
> be reluctant to get a medical evaluation because under [OSHA] the worker
> does not generally have transfer rights and wage retention rights.[35]

Finklea noted that the Federal Coal Mine Health and Safety Act is "the only law where we don't encounter these problems."[36] To control cancer in workers already exposed, Finklea asserted, steps must be taken to close the three gaps through which such cases now fall. We need a national health care system, improved worker's compensation systems, and a national job security program "that would require companies to find jobs in less hazardous areas for those employees that have been previously exposed."[37]

The backlog phenomenon may be unavoidable in occupational health. The more that is learned, the more often will mistakes of the past resurface. The worker who has been disabled as a result of risks he took unknowingly and without recompense may want assurances that he will be cared for and he and his family will be compensated as justly and fully as possible. But, the retrospective problem is serious for industry and for insurers, who have no good way of forecasting the future scope of the problem. Again, large firms are better equipped than smaller ones to handle an escalating or unpredictable compensation problem.

Still, it can be serious for any size firm. For example, on behalf of the asbestos industry, New Jersey Congresswoman Millicent H. Fenwick has filed legislation that would exempt companies from liability for deaths and disability from asbestosis or asbestos-linked lung cancer and provide federal compensation for affected workers. The nation's largest asbestos firm, Johns-Manville, is reportedly the defendant in nearly 400 lawsuits.[38] Labor and management are backing Fenwick's bill. An approach of this nature may be one workable approach to making restitution to victims of major occupational health disasters like asbestos. According to New Jersey Congressman Andrew McGuire, "approximately 1 million Americans are working with or have worked with asbestos. Of this group, an estimated 300,000 will die from some form of cancer."[39] Also, an amnesty program of some kind may be important to encourage generation of information about worksite health hazards:

> How do we set up a system so that the possessors of information have the incentives to collect it systematically and share it? We collectively are going to have to decide the level of investment to be made in obtaining information about these questions.
>
> Lee K. Benham

> I think the answer will be found in models from other areas where we have devised ways for dealing with the problem of liability. In transportation, for example, the National Transportation Safety Board and other groups involved in aviation have decided it's so important to find out why certain types of accidents and other events occur that they are willing to give absolute grants of immunity. Some activities of the Securities and Exchange Commission may also be models. We can draw from a variety of experiences in which we trade off certain types of liability immunity in order to obtain information that society badly needs.
>
> Paul M. Gertman

Both speakers seem to imply that irrespective of one's feelings about how much freedom workers have to chart their own destinies, broader societal issues are also at stake here.

Societal Trade-offs: Widening the Framework

Reduced to simplest terms, the occupational health problem is this: the high standard of living that industrialized nations have attained rests on many products that are hazardous to manufacture. Many of these products contribute to comfort and convenience, and some also to good health and longevity. But the production processes expose a relatively small segment of the population to a disproportionate share of the risk. In a few unequivocal cases, the logical solution may be removal of the offending substance from the workplace, as suggested by this exchange:

> Firemen and policemen are in inherently risky occupations that are recognized as such, and I wouldn't recommend getting rid of them. But in the asbestos industry I do not believe that it is fair to adjust for risk by paying a wage differential. For one thing, the pay differential firemen and policemen receive is a lot higher than anything the asbestos worker sees.
>
> Nicholas A. Ashford

Then it's a matter of price?

Richard H. Egdahl

Well, no. The point is the determination of whether the industry goes on or not—whether or not you need that industry for social reasons. That's the real question. Do we need to produce vinyl chloride—safely or unsafely? We need to put out fires—even if someone has to take risks to do it.

Dr. Ashford

Now we're widening the framework. This is the question we should be asking: Do we need this product in the first place?

Rick J. Carlson

In the vast majority of cases, Carlson's question will defy a simple answer; nor will it be obvious whose right it is to supply the answer. The products will have value and adequate and safe substitutes will be unavailable, prohibitively expensive, profligate of energy, or themselves conceivably as harmful as the more thoroughly tested substances they would replace. Modern technology is a two-edged sword, as eloquently stated by Barry Commoner in reference to the petrochemical industry, "that elegant new alchemy of our times":

> The petrochemical industry's products . . . make up a marvelous catalogue of useful materials . . . chemicals that can kill dandelions but not grass; repel mosquitoes, but not people; diminish sniffles, reduce blood pressure or cure tuberculosis . . . Yet the petrochemical industry dramatizes the paradox of modern technology: Its blessings are mixed with plagues.[40]

Commoner places hope in the Toxic Substances Control Act of 1976 because he believes it "can facilitate a discussion which will enable the people of the United States to decide how to respond to [this] sweeping challenge."[41]

In that public discussion, and in the others that will continue in this difficult area, more information, however qualified and flawed, will be better than less. Without wide dissemination of available information, along with a concerted effort to enrich the knowledge base, there will be little chance that decisions that are made will serve the broad public interest, even less that the public will perceive them so. With this observation, the volume comes full circle back to information about health services. There, as here, there are two basic and parallel themes: a need for better information and a need for fuller sharing of existing information with a more sophisticated public looking for common ground to participate—with the medical profession and with management—as informed partners sharing in the weighing of difficult decisions.

Summing Up

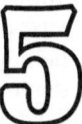

   The first volume in this series, which was both overview and preview of volumes to come, concluded that "private industry—both management and labor—plays a multidimensional and complex role in health care, with rising costs a precipitating factor and with concern for quality, equity, and access also very much in mind."[1] That role was divided into three parts:

> As a payer for health care on a large and growing scale through employee benefit packages, industry has vital interests that are tightly bound up with the nation's need to slow the rise of health care costs. As a provider of care through diverse in-house programs and clinics, industry faces dilemmas of accountability, confidentiality, and evaluation, along with expanded responsibilities for the health and welfare of workers. As a consumer of health care whose potential influence in the system derives in part from the massive numbers of workers who use health care services, industry has an opportunity and perhaps an obligation to share its expertise as well as to learn by participating in community efforts to find equitable ways to allocate limited resources and improve the quality of the health care system.[2]

This, the fourth volume in the series, has traced one central theme—the employee's expanding informational needs—through three successive topics in health, which can again be classified loosely in the three original categories. Physician advertising relates most directly to industry as a consumer of health care, HMO marketing to industry as purchaser, and occupational health communication to industry as provider of services to its own employees. The purpose of this volume has been to alert readers in industry and in health services to important changes now taking place in the environments in which their various roles in health are played.

Physician Advertising

Consumers of health care in the United States, the majority of whom are employees and their dependents, often lack useful information for deciding where to go for health services. The shortage of information has been caused in part by organized medicine's 131-year old ethical and professional codes, which are now undergoing both challenge and change. The codes originated in an era when the public probably needed protection from the wiles of the snake oil pitchman and huckster, but organized medicine's rules against solicitation of patients are believed by some to have outlived their usefulness. Encouraged by a series of court decisions, the Federal Trade Commission and consumer groups allege that the medical profession's control of the flow of information constitutes collusion and restraint of trade. As of this writing, the FTC investigation is still in adjudication and uncertainty remains concerning the impact of recent pertinent court decisions. But information concerning the medical profession seems likely to become increasingly available over the next several years.

What effect these changes will have on patients, and how far this ought to be pushed are controversial questions. Those who urge caution anticipate advertising chiefly by those physicians whose lack of skill or scruples explains their need to entice new patients. The profession, in this view, could be commercialized, physician-patient relationships compromised, health care costs elevated, and gullible patients harmed. In strong opposition is the view that suggests the profession has not volunteered information, and has thereby kept patients in ignorance about the health care system. The problem of health care costs is attributed by this group to market imperfections in health, which are, in turn, traced largely to the profession's embargo on information.

The wide middle ground is occupied by many—physicians and consumers alike—who foresee promise in physician advertising, but also potential pitfalls. They favor the release of more information than is now available, and worry less about self-serving claims by a few marginal practitioners than about whether the information provided will appear in a form that is intelligible and useful for consumers. They hope, therefore, that effective mechanisms can be developed for consumer groups to participate actively in the evaluation and dissemination of information about providers in the community.

Since health benefit plans administered by employers and unions are the financial access route to most of the health services consumed by employees, the question arises whether industry can fill the vacuum that now exists and assume a leadership role in collecting and evaluating needed information. A partial answer is offered by Willis B. Goldbeck, writing previously in this series:

> The myth that medical care providers are the only ones capable of understanding the medical care system must be overcome. Business and the providers can, and nearly always do, form a cooperative relationship. But for that relationship to have substance and durability, it must be based on the understanding that industry's role has changed from passive payer to active, informed participant.[3]

Marketing by Health Maintenance Organizations

Serving as a filter for information employees can use to select a personal physician is an unaccustomed activity for industry. But it relates conceptually to the role industry now plays in offering employees the option of joining a qualified HMO in lieu of traditional health insurance coverage. The mandatory dual choice provision of the Health Maintenance Organization Act of 1973 has given employers the opportunity to become a conduit of information for employees' decisions about where to go for health care.

Some employers who may not want to become involved in guiding their employees to individual providers in the community may be more comfortable with the idea of assisting them in the less subjective process of choosing a system of care. Differences between alternative systems can be difficult for employees to appraise, and they will often turn to the firm's benefits department as a convenient source of impartial information on the choice.

The federal government initiative, launched by the HMO Act, is being intensified by the Carter administration which recently called on the nation's industrial leaders for vigorous efforts to promote the growth of HMOs as a private sector approach to strengthening the market in health care and containing the rise in costs. HMOs have demonstrated the capacity to achieve significant economies, largely by substituting ambulatory care for hospitalization, and curtailing use of unneeded, high-technology diagnostic tests and therapies. Certainly not an instant answer to the problem of accelerating health care costs, HMOs do show some promise of slowing the rate of increase until it parallels the general economy.

Many large employers have by now offered at least one HMO option; substantial knowledge resides in industry about how HMOs operate and how to evaluate them. Corporations usually endeavor to present the HMO option in as neutral a light as possible, yet absolute neutrality is difficult to achieve and wide variability has been observed in the enthusiasm and support with which different firms greet an HMO's request for permission to market to employees. In geographic areas where the HMO concept is relatively unfamiliar, new plans face a major challenge putting their message across and often need all the help they can get. The degree to which industry becomes affirmatively involved in helping HMOs grow will probably make the difference in whether the movement can gather enough momentum soon enough to overcome a cost problem that is immediate and pressing.

Occupational Health Hazards

After a slow and painful period of initial implementation,[4] the Occupational Safety and Health Administration appears now to be moving forward to set comprehensive standards for occupational health hazards. Communicating with employees about hazards to which they have been exposed will increasingly be incorporated into management responsibilities, along with the general duty to provide a safe workplace. Communication serves as a kind of preventive medicine,[5] and is, in the case of real and present health hazards, generally acknowledged to be a crucial early step to take. As hazards become less immediate and not so easily discerned, however, consensus begins to dissipate. Discordant views of when and what management ought to communicate arise in part from differences of opinion concerning how much latitude employees truly have in deciding what risks they will assume on the job.

Chronic, low-level exposures to low probability risks present the thorniest problems of all for management policy. Here the extreme poles are occupied by, on one side, those contending that society should tolerate risky work only in the case of jobs that are essential for the common weal and that cannot be made safe. Otherwise, it is argued, individuals ought not to be put in the position of trading present financial security against a possible future illness, because the natural human response will be shortsighted when the danger seems remote. Opponents of this thinking credit the individual with sufficient judgment to make rational choices, given adequate information. But there are practical, scientific, and financial constraints on the availability of information about low-level health hazards in the workplace and these confound the issues related to communication.

The complexity of the challenge represented by occupational safety and health is underlined by the problems OSHA has experienced. OSHA's seven-year history, as well as the five-year history of the federal HMO program, demonstrate the limitations on federally legislated solutions to complex social problems. Goldbeck observed previously in this series that from industry's point of view, "government, more often than not, is an ally. New laws, regulations, and programs, however onerous, are also instruments of change which employers can turn to their advantage."[6]

The three legal developments that set the stage for this volume and the issues that emanate from them turn over the government-industry coin. Government clearly needs allies in the private sector to implement those new laws, regulations, and programs in ways that make the greatest sense for the people most directly affected.

Issues for the Future

The purpose of this chapter is to delineate an area in need of a creative dialogue. Its purpose should be to reassess the current in-house corporate health care delivery system and to identify the changes it should undergo if the country is to maintain safe and healthy workplaces at the most reasonable cost possible.

From the three basic topics of this volume—health professional advertising, HMO marketing, and employee information about occupational health—a unifying theme emerges. The issue of physician advertising raises questions about what information the employee can or cannot find about a health system that is external to his workplace. The same can be said about HMO marketing. On the other hand, informing the employee about his potential exposure to occupational health risks is an internal issue for industry and does not conceptually involve the external health care system. Or does it? This is the unifying theme. Should industry be working to strengthen the links between the health care of the employee at the workplace and his health care on the "outside"?

Unless this greater rapproachment between the two health care systems is confronted in a direct fashion, the current trend toward virtually complete separation will surely continue. And this trend may exact a terrible price in terms of duplication, confusion, and financial waste.

For a variety of reasons, industrial medicine has matured in a way that finds the industrial physician less a primary care practitioner than a specialist in safety and toxicology. This separation between medical care and occupational health in the United States is even more starkly and legally defined in some other countries such as Germany. But there are some strong reasons to reassess this traditional position.

Physician Advertising

In which environment is an employee likely to receive useful information about physicians and other aspects of the local external health care delivery system? In the present one, where the medical department's chief concern is occupational health as traditionally defined and the benefits department is saturated with daily demands that prevent it from counseling about alternatives for health care? Or a hypothetical one where a medical department is deeply involved in the range of employees' health problems and is up to date on various strengths and weaknesses of all the local health services and programs available to employees? Although the answer would seem obvious, there is little trend in the direction of having the industrial physician become involved in the primary care aspects of employee patients. Some notable exceptions, such as the Gillette plant in Boston, demonstrate that high-quality primary care medicine can be carried out in an industrial clinic, and that the same physicians who practice in industrial sites can practice in private offices, admit their patients to hospitals, and follow them as the responsible practitioners.

It is one thing to offer information furnished from the outside, but quite another to have the capabilities and assume the responsibility to filter that information to the employee and provide a critical analysis of it. We think it will be extremely difficult for an industry to provide a meaningful filter of health professional information that is being offered to employees without some involvement in health care delivery itself.

Advertising by HMOs

Under current circumstances, industries can decide whether to offer nonqualified HMOs to their employees, but they must offer qualified HMO plans. In most instances, the request by an HMO to be offered in the employee health benefit package is met with indifference or even hostility by the corporation, and in many cases a very small number of employees choose to join. Industry is simply purchasing something from the "outside" and is concerned with cost, reliability, and quality. This role provides little opportunity to "leverage" the system: it leaves industry to wait for the "external" health care world to make the offerings. If, on the other hand, industry were to become involved in some delivery of care to employees, it could instigate prepaid health plans either in combination with geographically dispersed fee-for-service physicians, or with corporate physicians themselves practicing in private offices part-time. To date, industry has for the most part not participated in the direct delivery of health care. We believe that this era is over and that industry will play an increasingly active partnership role with the private health delivery system in the care of employees.

This will also provide the basis for the development of some "hybrid" HMOs, which would build on the primary care capabilities of corporate clinics and include selected fee-for-service practicing physicians in the community. This form of industry-sponsored HMO might have great potential in areas where an industry has a large number of employees, and might provide competition to the conventional individual practice associations established by the county medical societies, on the one hand, and the salaried group HMO of the Kaiser variety, on the other.

In order for this to occur, the reporting relationships between the medical director and the industrial physicians under his charge must be very clear. There can be no question but that employees seen in the medical clinic of an industry are *patients*: their records must be kept confidential and the company must regard the medical department as sacrosanct.

Occupational Health Hazards

The third topic—reporting of information about occupational health hazards—also raises profound questions concerning the artificial separation between the "in-house" and "external" health care delivery systems. If employees are being subjected to toxic substances that will cause them harm, does it make sense to have the health care delivery system that will be treating them completely separate from the unit that diagnoses the condition and searches for its prevention? If it were accepted practice to have primary care physicians with expertise, not only in the toxicological and preventive aspects of occupational health diseases, but also in clinical diagnosis and therapy, the employee might be better served from the standpoint of his overall health care. Even in some large corporations, there is little communication among the benefits department, the medical director, and the industrial hygiene group.

There are some interesting possibilities for involving HMOs with occupational health problems. A further strengthening of ties between the in-house and external health care delivery systems could provide the basis for effective addition of OSHA's health challenges to the broader consideration of the employees' total health care needs.

The overriding challenge, then, is to evolve as specific a corporate strategy as possible on the appropriate role of primary medical care and health care delivery expertise and knowledge inside the corporation itself. There are many traditional reasons why this does not occur more frequently, but the increasingly stringent OSHA rules, combined with rising health care costs, have created an entirely new environment and set of imperatives. Traditionally, it has been difficult to get appropriately trained industrial physicians: very few medical schools even mention the topic. The time has come to reconsider the entire issue and explore the possibilities of thinking of attractive careers for entering medical students in industrial primary health care and occupational health. Unless we do so, and attack the problem along several fronts, including expansion of industrial primary care clinics, the training of professional health personnel capable of performing a wider range of tasks, providing intracorporate linkages between those responsible for OSHA and the medical department, and, most important, unless we have top management commitment to the effort, it will not occur.

Notes

Chapter 1

1. *Bates et al. v. State Bar of Arizona* (97 S. Ct. 2691).

2. Diana Chapman Walsh and Richard H. Egdahl, *Payer, Provider, Consumer: Industry Confronts Health Care Costs*, Springer Series on Industry and Health Care, no. 1 (New York: Springer-Verlag, Inc., 1977), pp. 1–45 (hereafter *Payer, Provider, Consumer*).

3. *The Health Maintenance Organization Act of 1973*, P.L. 93–222 (42 U.S.C. 300e Supp. IV, 1974).

4. *The Health Maintenance Organization Act Amendments of 1976*, P.L. 94–460 (42 U.S.C. 300e, ff.).

5. Department of Health, Education, and Welfare, Public Health Service, "Health Maintenance Organizations, Employees' Health Benefit Plans," *Federal Register*, 40 (208) (October 28, 1975): 50212–50216.

6. *The Occupational Safety and Health Act of 1970*, P.L. 91–596 (29 U.S.C. 651, ff.).

7. U.S. Congress, House, Manpower and Housing Subcommittee of the Committee on Government Operations, *Performance of the Occupational Safety and Health Administration: Hearings*, 91st Cong., 1st sess., April 27–28, 1977, p. 75 (hereafter *OSHA Hearings*, April 1977)

8. Ibid., p. 146.

9. *Payer, Provider, Consumer*, pp. 59–63.

10. Ibid., pp. 38–39.

11. Lee K. Benham, "Guilds and the Form of Competition in the Health Care Sector," U.S. Federal Trade Commission, Bureau of Economics, *Competition in the Health Care Sector: Past, Present and Future*, Proceedings of a Conference, June 1–2, 1977, ed. Warren Greenberg, in press (hereafter "Guilds and Competition").

12. *The Challenge of Consumerism: A Symposium* (New York: The Conference Board, 1971), p. 15.

13. Ibid., pp. 18–19.

14. Ibid., pp. 84–85.

15. Daniel S. Greenberg, "The Press and Health Care," *New England Journal of Medicine*, 297 (July 28, 1977); 231–232.

16. Ibid., p. 231.

Chapter 2

1. *Bates et al. v. State Bar of Arizona* (47 S. Ct. 2691).

2. Frank R. Stockton, "The Lady, or the Tiger?" in *An Anthology of Famous American Stories*, ed. Angus Burrell and Bennett Cerf (New York: Modern Library, 1953), pp. 248–253.

3. Ibid., p. 262.

4. Bonnie Bullough and Vern Bullough, "A Brief History of Medical Practice," in *Medical Men and Their Work*, ed. Eliot Friedson and Judith Lorber (Chicago: Aldine 1972), pp. 86–102.

5. E. S. Turner, *The Shocking History of Advertising* (New York: Dutton, 1953), p. 26.

6. Ibid.

7. Ibid., p. 84.

8. Quoted in ibid., p. 50.

9. American Medical Association, *Opinions and Reports of the Judicial Council* (Chicago, American Medical Association, 1971), p. iv.

10. Ibid., p. 22.

11. Abraham Flexner, *Medical Education in the United States and Canada* (New York: Carnegie Foundation for the Advancement of Teaching, Bulletin no. 4, 1910).

12. "Guilds and Competition."

13. William J. Bicknell and Diana Chapman Walsh, "Caveat Emptor: Exporting the U.S. Medical Model," *Social Science and Medicine*, 11 (1977): 285–288.

14. Walter Adams, ed., *The Structure of American Industry* (New York: MacMillan, 1977), p. vii.

15. David E. Rogers, "The Challenge of Primary Care," *Daedalus*, 106 (Winter 1977): 81–104.

16. Ibid., p. 86 (figure 2).

17. Ibid., p. 84.

18. Victor R. Fuchs, *Who Shall Live?* (New York: Basic Books, 1974), p. 60.

19. David Mechanic, "Approaches to Controlling the Costs of Medical Care," *New England Journal of Medicine*, 298 (5) (February 2, 1978): 249–254.

20. Ibid.

21. Michael J. Halberstam, "Professionalism and Health Care," in *Ethics of Health Care*, ed. Lawrence Tancredi (Washington, D.C.: National Academy of Sciences, 1974), p. 247.

22. Anne R. Somers and Herman M. Somers, "A Proposed Framework for Health and Health Care Policies," *Inquiry*, 14 (2) (June 1977): 161.

23. Alice M. Rivlin, Director, U.S. Congressional Budget Office, "Background Paper: Expenditures for Health Care: Federal Programs and their Effects" (August 1977), p. 57.

24. Alain C. Enthoven, "Consumer-Choice Health Plan," *New England Journal of Medicine*, 298 (12) (March 23 and March 30, 1978): 650–658, 709–720.

25. Max H. Parrott, Chairman, National Commission on the Costs of Medical Care, *Summary Report* (Chicago: American Medical Association, December 1977).

26. The Massachusetts Medical Society, "Synopsis and Proceedings of the Council Meeting October 12, 1977" (Boston: Massachusetts Medical Society, October, 1977), p. 29.

27. *Goldfarb v. State Bar*, 421, U.S. 773 (1975).

28. *Virginia Board of Pharmacy v. Virginia Citizens Consumer Council*, 425 U.S. 748 (1976).

29. *Bates et al. v. State Bar of Arizona* (47 S. Ct. 2691).

30. *Medical Care Review*, 34 (6) (1977): 627.

31. Richard H. Egdahl, et al., "The Potential of Organizations of Fee For Service Physicians for Achieving Significant Decreases in Hospitalization," *Annals of Surgery*, 186 (1977): 156–167.

32. Lee Benham, "The Effects of Advertising on the Price of Eyeglasses," *Journal of Law and Economics*, 15 (2) (October 1972): 337–352; Lee Benham and Alexandra Benham, "Regulating through the Professions: A Perspective on Information Control," *Journal of Law and Economics*, 18 (2) (October 1975): 421–447.

33. Quoted in "AMA, FTC Lawyers Clash as Trial Begins," *American Medical News* (September 12, 1977): 1.

34. Alan Booth and Nicholas Babchuk, "Seeking Health Care from New Resources," *Journal of Health and Social Behavior*, 13 (March 1977): 90–98.

35. Keith W. Sehnert, *How to Be Your Own Doctor (Sometimes)* (New York: Grosset and Dunlap, 1975).

36. Marvin S. Belsky and Leonard Gross, *How to Choose and Use Your Doctor* (New York: Fawcett World Library, 1976).

37. Donald M. Vickery and James F. Fries, *Take Care of Yourself: A Consumers' Guide to Health Care* (Reading, Mass.: Addison-Wesley, 1976).

38. Richard L. Peck, "Do the Yellow Pages Make You See Red?" *Medical Economics* (August 22, 1977): 114–118.

39. Ibid., p. 118.

40. *The Doctors Directory* (Tucson, Ariz.: Professional Guild of Arizona, June 1977).

41. *Directory of Evanston Primary Care Physicians* (Evanston, Ill.: Consumers' Health Group, Spring 1977).

42. Ibid., p. 7.

43. Keith W. Sehnert, *How to Be Your Own Doctor (Sometimes)* (New York: Grosset and Dunlap, 1975) p. 1.

44. "Chiropractic Advertising Attacked in Florida," *American Medical News* (October 31, 1977): 11.

45. "Clinics Sell 'A New You' in Want Ads," *American Medical News* (January 23, 1978): 11.

46. Richard Lewis, "AMA Continues Attack on Misleading M.D. Ads," *American Medical News* (January 23, 1978): 1, 11.

47. Dennis Connaughton, "The Turnabout on Physician Advertising," *American College of Surgeons Bulletin* (September 1977): 3.

48. Irvin Molotsky, "Dentists, Other Professionals Finding It Pays to Advertise," *New York Times* (January 17, 1978): 31.

49. Victor Cohn, "Doctors' Ads Tout Medical Bargains," *Washington Post* (November 28, 1977): A1.

50. Irvin Molotsky, "Dentists, Other Professions Finding It Pays to Advertise," *New York Times* (January 17, 1978): 31.

51. "AMA [American Management Association] Seminar Covers Aspects of Dental Plans: Trends, Designs, Costs, Premiums, Administration," *Employee Benefit Plan Review* (December 1977): 22.

52. "Unique Ad Strategy Increases Use of Sunrise Hospital on Weekends," *Federation of American Hospitals Review* (June 1977): 47.

53. Herman M. Somers, "The Malpractice Controversy and the Quality of Patient Care," *Milbank Memorial Fund Quarterly* (Spring 1977): 193.

54. "AMA [American Medical Association] Plans Advertising Campaign to Defeat 'Radical' National Health Insurance Plans," *NHI Reports* (November 7, 1977): 7.

55. Advertisment in the *Boston Globe* (December 30, 1977): 12.

56. Quoted in "FDA Begins Trial of MD Societies," *Medical World News* (September 19, 1977): 22.

57. Matt Clark, "Dr. Huckster," *Newsweek* (January 9, 1978): 70.

58. Ernest Gellhorn and William C. Canby, Jr., "Public and Private Restraints on Professional Advertising and Consumer Information," *Duke Law Journal* Symposium Issue on Antitrust Laws and the Health Services Industry, May, 1978, in press.

59. "Price Controllers are Reaching Out," *Business Week* (December 18, 1971): 31.

60. "FDA Begins Trial," *Medical World News* (September 19, 1977): 22.

61. Patrick O'Donoghue, *Evidence About the Effects of Health Care Regulation* (Denver, Colo.: Spectrum Research, 1974), p. 99.

62. Department of Health, Education and Welfare, "Health Planning National Guidelines," *Federal Register* 43 (March 28, 1978): 13040–13050.

Chapter 3

1. *Payer, Provider, Consumer*, pp. 30–33, 63–72.

2. "FTC Sues AMA Over Code of Ethics," *Science*, 197 (September 30, 1977): 1346.

3. Lawrence G. Goldberg and Warren Greenberg, "Staff Report on the Health Maintenance Organization and Its Effects on Competition" (Washington, D.C.: Federal Trade Commission, Bureau of Economics, July 1977).

4. Milton I. Roemer and William Shonick, "HMO Performance: The Recent Evidence," *Milbank Memorial Fund Quarterly: Health and Society*, 51 (Summer 1973): 271–317.

5. Frank H. Seubold, "HMOs: The View from the Program," *Public Health Reports*, 90 (1975): 99–103.

6. Paul M. Ellwood, Jr., et al., "Health Maintenance Strategy," *Medical Care*, 9 (1971): 291–298.

7. Paul Starr, "The Undelivered Health System," *Public Interest*, 42 (1976): 66–85.

8. U.S., Comptroller General, "Factors that Impede Progress in Implementing the Health Maintenance Organization Act of 1973: Report to the Congress," (Washington, D.C., HRD-76-128, September 3, 1976).

9. Richard McNeil, Jr., and Robert E. Schlenberg, "HMOs, Competition and Government," *Milbank Memorial Fund Quarterly: Health and Society* (Spring 1975): 195–224.

10. Clifton R. Gaus, Barbara S. Cooper, and Constance G. Hirshman, "Contrasts in HMO and Fee-for-Service Performance," *Social Security Bulletin* (May 1976): 3–14.

11. Lawrence G. Goldberg and Warren Greenberg, "Staff Report on the Health Mainte-

nance Organization and Its Effects on Competition" (Washington, D.C.: Federal Trade Commission, Bureau of Economics, July 1977).

12. Ibid., p. iv.

13. Richard H. Egdahl et al., "The Potential of Organizations of Fee for Service Physicians for Achieving Significant Decreases in Hospitalization," *Annals of Surgery*, 186 (1977): 156–167.

14. Lawrence Meyer, "Health Plans Grew in Seven Years, But Not as Much as Expected," *Washington Post* (January 3, 1978): 7a; "HMO Enrollment Up," *Group Health News*, 19 (January 1978): 1.

15. Frank H. Seubold, "HMOs: The View from the Program," *Public Health Reports*, 90 (1975): 99–103.

16. "What You Should Know About HMOs" (Washington, D.C.: U.S. Department of Health, Education, and Welfare, Publ. no. HSA–76–13039, 1976).

17. Arnold J. Rosoff, "Phase Two of the Federal HMO Development Program: New Directions After a Shakey Start," *American Journal of Law and Medicine*, 1 (2) (Fall 1975); 235 (note 98).

18. Carol N. D'Onofrio and Patricia Dolan Mullen, "Consumer Problems with Prepaid Health Plans in California," *Public Health Reports*, 92 (2) (March-April 1977): 121a

19. Reuben A. Kesel, "The AMA and the Supply of Physicians," *Law and Contemporary Problems* (Spring 1970): 251.

20. Everett M. Rogers and F. Floyd Shoemaker, *Communication of Innovations* (New York: Free Press, 1971).

21. Institute of Medicine, "Health Maintenance Organizations: Toward a Fair Market Test" (Washington, D.C.: National Academy of Sciences, 10M 74-03 May 1974).

22. Harold Magnuson, "The Right to Know," *Archives of Environmental Health* (January-February 1977): 41.

Chapter 4

1. Nicholas A. Ashford, *Crisis in the Workplace* (Cambridge, Mass.: MIT Press, 1976), p. 73.

2. Ibid.

3. Committee on Public Information in the Prevention of Occupational Cancer, "Informing Workers and Employers about Occupational Cancer" (Washington D.C.: National Academy of Sciences, 1977), pp. 23–24 (hereafter *PIPOC Report*).

4. Jean Seligmann, "Industrial Sterility," *Newsweek* (August 29, 1977): 69.

5. U.S. Department of Health, Education, and Welfare, *Report of the HEW Secretary's Commission on Pesticides and Their Relationship to Environmental Health* (1969), p. 568.

6. "Guidelines on Pregnancy and Work," and "Comprehensive Bibliography on Pregnancy and Work," (Chicago, Ill.: American College of Obstetricians and Gynecologists, 1976).

7. Leon J. Warshaw, "The Pregnant Worker," *Journal of Occupational Medicine* (in press).

8. James C. Hyatt, "Early Warning: Protection for Unborn? Work Safety Issue Isn't As Simple as it Sounds," *Wall Street Journal*, Tuesday, August 16, 1977, p. 1.

9. *Preventive Medicine USA*: Task Force Reports Sponsored by the John E. Fogarty International Center for Advanced Study in the Health Sciences, National Institutes of Health, and the American College of Preventive Medicine (New York: Prodist, 1976), pp. 540–552.

10. William W. Lowrance, *Of Acceptable Risk:* Science and the Determination of Safety (Los Altos, Calif.: William Kaufmann, Inc., 1976).

11. Panel on Chemicals and Health of the President's Science Advisory Committee, *Chemicals and Health* (Washington, D.C.: Science and Technology Policy Office, National Science Foundation, September 1973), p. 131.

12. Ibid., p. 11.

13. U.S. Code of Federal Regulations 409 (c) (3) (A), and 512 (d) (1) (H).

14. President's Advisory Committee, *Chemicals and Health*, p. 131.

15. Ibid., p. 29.

16. *Preventive Medicine USA*, p. 544.

17. John T. Talty, "Carcinogens in Industry," Letter to the Editor, *Science*, 198 (October 28, 1977): 354.

18. Thomas H. Maugh II, "Carcinogens in the Workplace: Where to Start Cleaning Up," *Science* 197 (September 23, 1977): 1268–1269.

19. "The Right to Know: Practical Problems and Policy Issues Arising from Exposures to Hazardous Chemical and Physical Agents in the Workplace," Policy paper prepared by the National Institute for Occupational Safety and Health (Rockville, Md.: Center for Disease Control, July 1977).

20. Committee on Public Information in the Prevention of Occupational Cancer, National Academy of Sciences, "Public Information in the Prevention of Occupational Cancer: Proceedings of a Symposium," December 2–3, 1976 (Springfield, Va.: National Technical Information Service, April 1977), (hereafter *PIPOC Proceedings*).

21. Ibid., p. 147–176.

22. Ibid., p. 147.

23. OSHA Hearings, April 1977, p. 66.

24. Ibid., p. 146.

25. "Health Records Face a Privacy Challenge," *Business Week* (October 31, 1977): 38.

26. The Privacy Protection Study Commission, *Personal Privacy in an Information Society* (Washington, D.C.: U.S. Government Printing Office [stock no. 052-003-00395-3,], July 1977).

27. "Health Records and Privacy: What Would Hippocrates Say?" *Science*, 198 (October 28, 1977): 382.

28. Alan F. Westin, *Computers, Health Records, and Citizen Rights* (Washington, D.C.: U.S. Government Printing Office [stock no. 003-003-0168-1], 1976), p. 1.

29. "Health Records and Privacy: What Would Hippocrates Say?" *Science*, 198 (October 28, 1977): 382.

30. William E. Morton, "The Responsibility to Report Occupational Health Risks," *Journal of Occupational Medicine*, 19 (April 1977): 258–260.

31. Albert L. Nichols and Richard Zeckhauser, "Government Comes to the Workplace: An Assessment of OSHA," *The Public Interest*, 49 (February 1977): 39–69.

32. David Burnham, "Agency Plan to Identify and Control Toxic Chemicals Arouses a Dispute," *New York Times* (March 5, 1978), p. 1, 46.

33. Ibid., p. 46.

34. Margot Hornblower, "Placing Dollar-and-Cent Value on Life," *Washington Post* (November 7, 1976) p. 1.

35. *OSHA Hearings*, April 1977, p. 49.

36. Ibid.

37. Ibid., p. 53.

38. "Asbestos Firms Seek Way Out of Lawsuits," *Boston Globe* (October 1977), p. 12.

39. U.S. Congress, House, Subcommittee on Oversight and Investigations of the Committee on Interstate and Foreign Commerce, *Environmental Causes of Cancer: Hearings,* 94th Cong., 2d. sess., May 28 and September 20, 1976, p. 2.

40. Barry Commoner, "The Promise and Perils of Petrochemicals," *New York Times Magazine* (September 25, 1977): 38.

41. Ibid., p. 73.

42. Robert Stewart Smith, *The Occupational Safety and Health Act: Its Goals and Its Achievements* (Washington, D.C.: American Enterprise Institute for Public Policy Research, 1976).

Chapter 5

1. *Payer, Provider, Consumer,* p. 91.

2. Ibid., p. 2.

3. Willis. B. Goldbeck, *A Business Perspective on Industry and Health Care,* Springer Series on Industry and Health Care, no. 2. (New York: Springer-Verlag, 1978), p. 50 (hereafter *Business Perspective*).

4. U.S. Congress, House, Committee on Government Operations, "Failure to Meet Committments Made in the Occupational Safety and Health Act," 95th Cong., 1st sess. (House Report no. 95–710), October 17, 1977.

5. Brenda L. Dervin, in *PIPOC Proceedings,* p. 109.

6. *Business Perspective,* p. 49.

BACKGROUND PAPERS

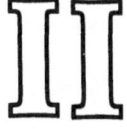

Advertising by Health Care Professionals: Issues and Prospects

Ronald Stiff and Paul N. Bloom

7

The recent Supreme Court decision (*Bates et al. v. State Bar of Arizona*) allowing limited forms of price advertising by lawyers—and the wave of advertising by lawyers and other professionals that followed—has created a sense of urgency about the need to resolve how and where professionals should be permitted to advertise. The health care professions are heavily involved in this controversy. The Federal Trade Commission is attempting to have the American Medical Association's rules prohibiting advertising declared anti-competitive, while a variety of other actions have been initiated by the government or private individuals to remove bans against advertising by dentists, ophthalmologists, and other health care professionals.

In general, the pro-advertising forces argue that advertising would lead to more competition among providers and more cost-effective services, citing studies that found the prices of eyeglasses and prescription drugs to be significantly lower in states where advertising is permitted.[1] However, these are tangible goods; there is a strong possibility that different, less favorable outcomes might occur for intangible services. A careful examination of the potential effects of permitting advertising by health care professionals is therefore needed before a final policy determination is made.

Potential Types of Advertising

Our environment is already saturated with health care communications. For instance, Smith et al. monitored a week of television broadcasting and found that about 7 percent of all commercial and program broadcast time contained health-related content.[2] Additionally, health information is available from public health agencies, the printed news media, communications at the workplace, and personal interactions with health care professionals. It therefore seems likely that the consumer will respond only to advertising by health care professionals that provides new information.

These new messages are likely to be designed as specific cues to action. Those from primary care providers will attempt to cue such actions as establishing a relationship with a provider, seeking preventive care, or seeking symptomatic care. Secondary care professionals are most likely to concentrate on cues to seek symptomatic care, while other providers (including nurses and paraprofessionals) may originate cues to seek preventive care.

The media used for advertising are likely to be somewhat limited, even in the absence of legal barriers to media choice. The cues to action suggested are fairly complex and consequently lend themselves to printed advertisements. Health care services are also by their nature geographically bound—encouraging the use of local newspaper advertising say, for encouraging people to join an HMO or to utilize a particular coronary care facility. Only a cue with wide appeal to take a very simple preventive action (such as immunization or a simple test) can be transmitted effectively through radio and television.

Thus far, the Supreme Court has ruled only on the First Amendment legality of price advertising of prescription drugs and price advertising of routine services by attorneys in the print media, expressing a clear intention to proceed slowly and cautiously on the issue of advertising by professionals. For example, further rulings beyond *Bates v. State Bar of Arizona* will be needed to determine whether lawyers can make "quality" claims in their advertisements, use in-person or indirect solicitation of clients, or place advertisements in the broadcast media.

Although it may take quite some time before the court considers the health care professions, it seems reasonably clear based on the *Virginia Pharmacy Board v. Virginia Consumer Council* and *Bates* decisions that price advertising of routine services in the print media by doctors and other health care professionals cannot be legally restricted. It also seems reasonably clear that the advertising of basic factual information such as name, address, specialty, telephone number, and office hours in the print media will be permitted. What is not clear, however, is how "routine" services and "basic factual information" will be defined.

In *Bates* the court found "uncontested divorces," "uncontested bankruptcies", and "changes of name" to be routine legal services. But three of the four dissenting justices expressed deep concern about the possibility that deception would occur in price advertising of even these services. They feared that people might go to a lawyer because of his or her low price for a routine service, and then find that their needs were not routine and would cost more to serve than they expected.

From this concern one can anticipate a rather narrow definition of "routine" services and "basic factual information" in all the professions. Nevertheless, health care professionals should still be able to advertise the prices for a large number of services (simple surgical procedures, examinations) and list a large number of facts about themselves (degrees, board certifications, honors, languages spoken, payment plans accepted) in advertisements. One can expect a "glossary of acceptable terms to use in health care advertising" to appear— perhaps developed by the American Medical Association with the approval of the antitrust enforcement agencies and the Supreme Court.

It is extremely difficult to predict how much freedom health care professionals will ultimately have in the three decision-making areas that were not covered in the *Bates* decision. A likely outcome would be for the court to allow restrictions against "quality" claims to remain—in order to protect consumers who do not have the skills to know which of several "best" doctors is really the best—but to eliminate restrictions against in-person solicitation and against broadcast advertisements that merely present prices of "routine" services or "basic factual information."

There is a possibility that *all* restrictions against advertising by health care professionals could be declared illegal if the courts are convinced they are in violation of the antitrust laws. However, the chances of such a ruling are slim, since many of the existing restrictions against advertising are insulated from antitrust liability under the *Parker v. Brown* doctrine, which allows violations of the antitrust laws if expressly directed by a state government. Only in those states where health care advertising restrictions have not been approved by the state could an antitrust violation be found. (One such is Connecticut where the FTC is pursuing its case against the American Medical Association and its state and local affiliates). Furthermore, in these states it would not be surprising to see health care professionals lobby for and obtain legislation to allow certain advertising restrictions to receive *Parker v. Brown* protection.

Potential Effects of Permitting Advertising

Assuming that health care professionals will be allowed to advertise the prices of "routine" services and "basic factual information" in all media, how will society be affected? Who will advertise? How will consumers respond? And how will advertising affect competition among providers and, consequently, their fees and services?

Extent of Provider Advertising

In the absence of legal or professional sanctions, the amount of advertising done will depend primarily upon the supply and demand conditions within various specialties. The typical overburdened provider could not be expected to advertise unless he believed that doing so would improve the effectiveness of this practice in some way other than by increasing the number of patients. He might, for example, want to use advertising to educate patients to seek care at the most appropriate time contingent upon their symptoms. However, this form of advertising is unlikely to occur since it would be similar to many existing health care communications and have limited effectiveness. Moreover, if the advice offered in an educational advertisement could be questioned by other competent professionals, a provider's reputation and practice could be severely damaged.

We must therefore conclude that advertising would only tend to be used by underutilized providers, such as new practices and large HMOs. Underutilization can also occur when supply in a specialty exceeds demand, as is the case with certain secondary care dentists and physicians. An underutilized cardiologist, for example, could encourage weekend athletes over forty to visit for preactivity evaluations. Finally, paramedics, nurses, dental hygienists, and others may perceive advertising as a means of building a practice of their own.

Consumer Response to Advertising

Consumers have been shown to respond to some fairly unusual forms of medical "information." For example, a rancher who had cancer chose self-treatment with "chaparrel tea" over surgery. The tea was widely reported in the press as an actual or potential cure, producing over 14,000 letters, cables, and telephone calls and even some patient referrals. Based on experiences like this, Reemtsma and Maloney have proposed a law: "The public impact of instant medical reporting is related inversely to the intrinsic merit of the observation."[3]

Unlike the chaparrel tea news story, advertising by health care professionals will generally be mundane in content and may often be mundane in effect. We need to evaluate whether consumers will use advertisements for selection of primary care providers, whether they will do more comparison shopping, and whether consumer self-referrals to secondary care providers will increase. We might also ask whether consumers will become more discriminating in their response for care, especially for preventive care and whether they will be misled by advertisements.

Research has shown (in England) that selection of a primary care provider is generally casual, with little consideration of physician qualifications.[4] Most consumers selected the nearest physician or one used by a relative or friend. Booth and Babchuk found consumers seeking new health care providers seldom recalled consulting with more than one person.[5] Most consumers made their selections in less than two months, although the elderly and lower socio-economic strata reported both fewer interpersonal communications and greater delay in establishing resources. The generally casual selection decision may occur because consumers consider all professionals offering similar services to be acceptably competent. A very simple cue from either a friend or an advertisement may therefore be sufficient to create a response when a need exists. The use of advertisements as a cue may be even more acceptable to the poor and elderly who have few interpersonal resources.

Moreover, if consumers begin to shop more seriously for primary care and seek larger amounts of helpful information, they could begin to use advertisements even more. In fact, the findings of Kasteler et al. suggest that some more serious shopping is already taking place. Nearly half their respondents reported that they had doctor-shopped within the past year. This behavior was initiated by dissatisfaction with either technical competence or socio-emotional factors.[6]

While an expected increase in doctor-shopping should lead to more usage of advertising, it is not immediately clear whether the reverse is also true. Of course, the proponents of advertising firmly believe that comparison shopping *would* increase with the availability of advertising, as it would reduce consumer search costs. However, this may occur in shopping for primary care and preventive care and not in shopping for secondary care. Consumer self-referral to secondary care physicians seems to be quite limited: Shortell reports that fewer than 11 percent of the referrals to secondary care physicians were patient initiated.[7] Advertising is unlikely to be a more powerful persuader than the advice of one's own primary physician, and it is also unlikely that the highly specific and individualized link between specific symptoms and qualified specialists could be adequately communicated through an advertisement.

On the other hand, greater discrimination by consumers, and therefore more use of advertising and more comparison shopping, may be possible in relation to preventive care—which can be planned with less urgency and physical risk. For example, Breslow and Somers propose a lifetime health monitoring program with specific procedures and tests for ten different age groups.[8] Many health care professionals and paraprofessionals could provide these procedures and tests at reasonable prices, and advertising could probably help them obtain enough patients to survive financially.

Clearly, there is a risk that those who provide preventive care—or any other type of health care services, for that matter—could mislead consumers through their advertising. Deception could occur even if the "glossary of acceptable advertising terms" is very carefully designed. Close monitoring by the FTC, local consumer protection agencies, and professional associations will therefore be needed to control the amount of misleading information that appears. However, as time goes on and consumers become more familiar with the content of health care advertising, the need for strong protective measures will diminish.

Effects on Competition, Fees, and Services

If moderate amounts of primary care and preventive care advertising are indeed done and used by consumers in comparison shopping, competition among these providers should increase and should produce some lowering of fees, increased cost-effectiveness, and greater service variety.

Lower fees could come about in several ways. First, price advertising could bring on some price rivalry, but only for standardized, routine services that could have their prices readily advertised. Price advertising for more complex, nonroutine services would probably be restricted and, even if allowed, would probably not be effective in attracting the many consumers who have health insurance available to pay for nonroutine primary care services.

Lower fees for *all* types of primary care and preventive care services could also come about as a result of competitive pressures produced by advertising in making it easier for group primary care practices, HMOs, and paraprofessionals offering preventive care services (such as physical therapy or teeth cleaning) to attract consumers. Others could potentially use advertising to ease their entry into certain markets and to help build practices of more cost efficient sizes. Eventually, competitive and, perhaps, regulatory pressures would allow the lower costs achieved by these more optimally sized practices to be passed on to consumers. In addition, emphasis by more of these practices on preventive care might eventually lead to a lowering of overall costs, to the extent that serious illnesses could be forestalled.

Competitive pressures might also enhance the quality of services and would give consumers a much wider variety of providers to choose from. Advertising might accelerate the growth of group practices that use some paraprofessionals and seem to operate effectively.[9] For example, Shortell has found that group practices are more likely to refer patients to specialists.[10] Another way health care quality might improve is if a desire to look superior in advertising leads many professionals to compete with one another by obtaining new certifications and other new credentials.

Thus, advertising would tend to produce several favorable results by, among other things, easing entry into certain health care markets. It seems highly unlikely that advertising would, instead, produce the reverse effect of further raising entry barriers and injuring competition. Theoretically, it could do so by creating loyalty for certain providers or by producing significant cost advantages for large advertisers over small advertisers. But the amount of advertising that would be done in health care would probably not be large enough to allow these types of outcomes to occur. Furthermore, there is considerable doubt among many scholars whether *any* amount of advertising can create brand loyalty or significant cost advantages.[11]

The possible effects of advertising on the delivery of secondary care are hard to forecast. With little advertising expected by secondary providers, direct effects on competition, fees, or types of services seem unlikely. Advertising could, however, have indirect effects on how secondary care is provided. For example, if primary care providers are compelled by competitive pressures to be more selective in choosing their referral networks, secondary care providers might start to compete more vigorously on a price or quality basis to get into the referral networks of the prosperous and prestigious primary care providers.

Conclusions

We have predicted that advertising by health care professionals would probably lead to more competition, lower fees, higher quality care, and more varieties of care within certain health care specialties. These results would probably occur for providers of primary care and preventive care, but not necessarily for secondary care providers.

Of course, advertising could only produce these forecasted results if it were legal, if it were used by primary care and preventive care providers, and if consumers actually used it to help them choose such providers. Future empirical research on these assertions could be done effectively using a quasi-experimental approach, comparing the experience of the first states that permit health care advertising as experimental groups with that of laggard states as control groups.

NOTES

1. Lee Benham, "The Effects of Advertising on the Price of Eyeglasses," *Journal of Law and Economics* 15:337–352 (October 1972); and John F. Cady, *Drugs on the Market* (Lexington, Mass.: Lexington Books, 1975).

2. Frank A. Smith, Geoffrey Trivax, David A. Zuehlke, Paul Lowinger, and Thieu L. Nghiem, "Health Information during a Week of Television," *New England Journal of Medicine* 286:516–520 (March 9, 1972).

3. Keith Reemtsma and James V. Maloney, Jr., "The Economics of Instant Medical News," *New England Journal of Medicine* 290:439–442 (February 21, 1974).

4. Ann Cartwright, *Patients and Their Doctors: A Study of General Practice* (New York: Atherton, 1967).

5. Alan Booth and Nicholas Babchuk, "Seeking Health Care from New Resources," *Journal of Health and Social Behavior* 13:90–99 (March 1972).

6. Josephine Kasteler, Robert L. Kane, Donna M. Olsen, and Constance Thetford, "Issues Underlying Prevalence of 'Doctor-Shopping' Behavior," *Journal of Health and Social Behavior* 17(4):328–339 (Dec., 1976).

7. Stephen M. Shortell, *A Model of Physician Referral Behavior: A Test of Exchange Theory in Medical Practice*, University of Chicago, Center of Health Administration Studies, Research Series, no. 31 (1972).

8. Lester Breslow and Anne R. Somers, "The Lifetime Health-Monitoring Program," *New England Journal of Medicine* 296:601–608 (March 17, 1977).

9. Eugene C. Nelson, Arthur R. Jacobs, Karyn Cordner, and Kenneth G. Johnson, "Financial Impact of Physician Assistants on Medical Practice," *New England Journal of Medicine* 293:527–530 (September 11, 1975); and Fred E. Graham, "Group versus Solo Practice: Arguments and Evidence," *Inquiry* 9:49–60 (June 1972).

10. Shortell et al., *Physician Referral Behavior*.

11. James M. Ferguson, *Advertising and Competition: Theory, Measurement, Fact* (Cambridge, Mass.: Ballinger, 1974).

The Consumer Comes First in Professional Advertising

Emlyn I. Griffith and Frank C. Abbott

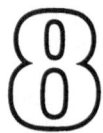

In New York State, the Board of Regents recently completed a codification of rules defining unprofessional conduct. This paper describes the development of these rules, particularly as they relate to professional advertising—a development that will lead to far-reaching changes in the communication between practitioner and patient.

For many years in New York, as in most states, statutes virtually prohibited advertising in the health professions. The new rules attempt to distinguish between factual advertising which gives useful information and purely commercial advertising which seeks to promote a particular practitioner; they permit the former and restrict the latter. To understand the new rules, some background is needed in the regulation of the professions in New York State, the process by which the rules have been developed, and the manner in which they will influence practice.

New York's System of Professional Governance

Unlike any other state, New York has an umbrella system of professional governance. The state's Education Department is responsible under the Board of Regents for the education, licensure, and discipline of virtually all learned professions except law and theology—thirty in number. These functions are administered by an Education Department staff of more than 200 persons. Advisory professional boards are appointed by the Regents, with specific duties to assist them and the Department in professional licensing and practice, including hearing and determining charges of misconduct. The Regents are authorized to issue rules and to approve regulations promulgated by the commissioner of education for the governance of the professions. Such rules and regulations have the force of law.

From Proposal to Regulations: A Year of Controversy

After the Board of Regents determined that its rules defining unprofessional conduct should be reviewed, updated, and codified, and under a mandate perceived as the first-of-its kind Conference on the Professions in New York City on November 18, 1975, a composite draft defining unprofessional conduct was ready for review in December 1976. Several drafts, public hearings and Regents meetings later, the rules were adopted on July 28, 1977. They became effective on October 1, 1977.

In this entire process, the most controversial section was the rule on advertising. Many, but not all, professions were comfortable with their protected status "removed from any commercial temptations." Most consumer groups were aligned on the other side; indeed, some had initiated law suits against the Regents over enforcement of the existing rules restricting professional advertising.

Initial proposals defined as unprofessional conduct any "advertising . . . that is not in the public interest." They proceeded to cite several acceptable forms of advertising, including bidding on public contracts, listing in directories, etc. Price advertising was not included and a substantial burden was placed on the licensee to defend his or her action in any dubious advertisement.

No rules were more debated at the public hearings that followed than those affecting advertising. Consumer advocates, public and private, argued that "advertising regulations should be limited to the traditional forms of prohibitions, such as false and misleading advertising or bait-and-switch advertising . . . This section of the proposed rules is wholly inadequate to the needs of consumers and the trend of court pronouncements." The professional societies and professional boards, on the other hand, counseled against relaxation of regulations and felt, in addition, that the wording of the proposed rule was so vague as to have no practical meaning. Medical, dental, and podiatry societies were the most strongly opposed. However, discussions emphasized that, different as were their perspectives, all participants were concerned about the best interest of the public.

In the next draft of the proposal, the Regents shifted the approach from a general prohibition of "advertising not in the public interest" to a specific enumeration of proscribed activities and approaches.

After a public hearing in May 1977 and additional written comment from interested societies and agencies, the Regents in late June reviewed a near-final version of the proposed rules that some society representatives regarded as too liberal and some consumer agency representatives regarded as still too restrictive. In these rules, "advertising or soliciting for patronage that is not in the public interest" was defined as unprofessional conduct. This concept was further defined to include advertising that is false, fraudulent, deceptive, misleading, sensational, or flamboyant; involves intimidation or undue pressure; utilizes testimonials; guarantees a service; offers free services or discounts on professional services; or makes claims of professional superiority that the licensee cannot substantiate.

Listing prices for professional services, as distinguished from articles or goods, was also defined as unprofessional conduct. Two exceptions were that prices for specific professional services could be included in "professional directories published by third parties which are open without charge to all members of the profession practicing in the geographic area covered by the directories" and that for the health professions, such prices could be stated in information provided to members of group health plans.

The Regents were anticipating a decision by the United States Supreme Court in a lawyer advertising case, and three days later it came. On Monday, June 27, the decision in *Bates et al. v. State Bar of Arizona* was handed down by the high court, prompting reexamination by the Regents' committees of proposals that would have limited strictly the advertising of fees for services: should they remove all restrictions on price advertising, leave their proposals unchanged, or adopt an intermediate position?

A bit of drama was inevitable on July 27, as members of the Regents' committees went to work on the final draft of the rules prior to formal action by the two committees and the entire board the next day. A press briefing had been arranged for the morning of July 28, and a press conference was scheduled for the afternoon following board action. The proposed rules were unique in the nation, and the *Bates* decision had stimulated media interest. The Committees on Higher and Professional Education and Professional Discipline, meeting that Wednesday evening, hammered out their final position. By midnight, the concepts were clear and the language in place, subject only to a final review the next morning.

The approved wording held closely to the positions taken by the Supreme Court in *Bates*. The New York regulation now states: "The following shall be deemed appropriate means of informing the public of the availability of professional services: ... the advertising in a newspaper, periodical or professional directory of fixed prices, or a stated range of prices, for specified routine professional services, provided such advertisement clearly states whether additional charges may be incurred for related services which may be required in individual cases."

Together with the remaining subsections of the rule, this language has the effect of permitting professional advertising, other than the prices of professional services, in all media and by other devices such as signs, letterheads, and cards, provided it does not contravene the prohibitions against false, misleading, and flamboyant advertising. Advertising of fees for professional services will be limited, however, to the print media, to services that are specific and routine, and to prices that are fixed or of a stated range.

In the *Bates* decision, the Supreme Court majority held its determination to the facts at hand and specifically excepted from the scope of its decision the issue of advertising in the broadcast media. The Regents similarly limited their rule on price advertising, prohibiting it on television and radio.

In adopting the rules the Regents acknowledged that: "A period of practice under the new Rules should provide for experience that will demonstrate gains and, possibly, losses from the standpoint of the well-being of the public. Where it appears after a reasonable period of time that changes should be made, the Regents clearly will make them."

Enforcing the New Regulation

The very structure of Regents' governance of the professions helps to assure equitable, even-handed application of the rules defining unprofessional conduct to the nearly half million registered professionals in New York. Both the public and the professional boards noted above are involved. The boards exercise key roles in application of the rules, and their members are aware of both their primary duty to protect the public and a concomitant duty to assist practitioners.

Any report or complaint of unprofessional conduct is directed to the Education Department, whose investigators obtain the evidence that will lead either to the voting of charges or to dismissal of the complaint. The evidence is referred to a screening panel composed of three members of the state board for the appropriate profession which determines whether formal charges should be drawn. If so, the file is referred to the Attorney General's Education Bureau in New York City where the charges are drawn and a hearing is scheduled.

The panel for the formal hearing is composed of five members of the state board for the profession of the practitioner being charged. Thus, at both the screening and hearing stages, professionals of experience and stature are involved.

At the same time, the general public is well represented in the process. The Education Department has no allegiance to any particular profession; nor do the Regents, fifteen lay persons elected by the state Legislature. Significantly, the process of determining guilt or innocence starts with the peer group but ends with the Regents. The peer group only *recommends* to the Regents.

After the formal hearing by the peer group, the Regents Review Committee conducts its own review hearing based upon the record of the peer group hearing, with the respondent present, usually accompanied by counsel. This committee may modify findings within the record, but it is primarily concerned with affirming or modifying the measure of discipline recommended by the peer group if the respondent was found guilty. Review Committee recommendations in turn are reviewed by the Regents, acting through their standing Committee on Professional Discipline, and finally adopted by the full board.

The procedure, which is usually completed within sixty days from recommendation by the peer panel to final action by the Regents, provides checkpoints manned by department officers and regents. There is ongoing review of the activities of the professional peer groups from consideration of evidence and voting of charges to findings and penalty recommendations. Final determinations rest with the Regents. The system assures consideration of factors unique to the practice of any profession and, at the same time, assures governance by a lay board responsible to the general public, not to any individual or professional group.

The consumer *should* come first in professional advertising. Public interest has been the baseline for every decision of the Regents in developing the new rules—often in the face of vigorous, honest contention among professional and consumer groups, especially in regard to fee advertising.

Recent court decisions, in concert with the Regents' rules, will open new avenues of communication for professionals and the public. For the consumer, these new avenues may solve some old problems and may create some new problems. If the advantages outweigh the disadvantages, then the effort will have been worthwhile.

Regardless of the ultimate outcome and the judgment of history, the New York Regents can say they tried. They have recognized changing conditions, identified serious problems, and proposed realistic solutions. In their concern for consumers they are exercising both a statutory duty and a public trust.

Appendix

Rules of the New York State Board of Regents Relating to Definitions of Unprofessional Conduct

Section 29.1 General provisions for all professions.

(b) Unprofessional conduct in the practice of any profession licensed or certified pursuant to Title 8 of the Education Law shall include:
. . .
  (12) Advertising or soliciting for patronage that is not in the public interest.
    i) Advertising or soliciting not in the public interest shall include but not be limited to advertising that:
      1) Is false, fraudulent, deceptive, misleading, sensational, or flamboyant.
      2) Represents intimidation or undue pressure.
      3) Uses testimonials.
      4) Guarantees any service.
      5) Offers gratuitous services or discounts in connection with professional services, but this clause shall not be

construed to relate to the negotiation of fees between professionals and patients or clients, or to prohibit the rendering of professional services for which no fee is charged.

6) Makes claims of professional superiority which cannot be substantiated by the licensee, who shall have the burden of proof.

7) States or includes prices for professional services, except as provided for in section 29.1 (b) (12) ii) 2), below.

      ii) The following shall be deemed appropriate means of informing the public of the availability of professional services:

        1) Informational advertising not contrary to the foregoing prohibitions.

        2) The advertising in a newspaper, periodical or professional directory of fixed prices, or a stated range of prices, for specified routine professional services, provided such advertisement clearly states whether additional charges may be incurred for related services which may be required in individual cases.

The Availability of Health Information

George R. Dunlop

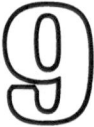

Today it is becoming increasingly difficult for consumers to select a physician properly. In every large city, thousands enter the health care system through emergency wards, simply because they know no better way. The contributing factors are the mobility of our society, the increasing density of population in larger cities, and the fragmentation and depersonalization of the medical care process.

To date, most of the information available to the public on how to select a physician is found in lay periodicals. Articles on how consumers should evaluate physicians have appeared recently in *Ladies Home Journal*,[1] *Good Housekeeping*,[2] and *Newsweek*.[3] Addressing the same problem, *Consumer Reports*[4] has described how to develop a directory of physicians. Public officials have also provided some information. Pennsylvania's one-time insurance commissioner published a series of *Shopper's Guides*, to hospitals, to health insurance, to dentistry, and to surgery.[5] Notable for its absence from the list of those providing this trickle of information is the medical profession, although

at least one study has concluded that there is in fact no information deficit—
that most physicians will answer consumers' questions over the phone.[6]

Public attention has recently been drawn to this issue by the actions of
the Federal Trade Commission and the Supreme Court.[7] The FTC has charged
the American Medical Association, the Connecticut State Medical Society, and
the New Haven County Medical Association with "anticompetitive actions,"
and proposes to require them to loosen their strictures on advertising. The
AMA replies that it approves of legitimate advertising, including fee information, but forbids solicitation of patients. "Solicitation," as defined by the AMA,
is inherently deceptive: it is the attempt to gain patients through testimonials,
inflated self-laudatory claims, or falsehoods.

However, societies are already reluctant to take action against such
deceptive advertising because of the United States Supreme Court's 1977
decision in *Bates et al. v. State Bar of Arizona.*[8] The court concluded that states
may not prevent the publication in a newspaper of truthful advertisement
concerning the availability and terms of routine legal services. The court's
opinion rests on the unsupported assumption that lawyers—and therefore,
presumably, physicians, although this is yet to be decided—will not advertise
anything but "routine" services, which the court totally fails to define, or if
they do advertise more, that the profession and the courts will be able to protect
the public from the few practitioners who abuse their trust. But the existing
administrative machinery of both the medical profession and the courts has
already proved wholly inadequate to police the profession effectively.

To be sure, the public needs information concerning physicians, their
work and their fees, but at the same time the public needs protection from the
unscrupulous and incompetent practitioner anxious to prey on the uninformed. It seems that these twin goals can best be served by permitting
organized medicine to experiment with and perfect programs that would
announce to the public the probable range of fees for specifically defined
services and thus give patients some idea of the potential cost when seeking
medical assistance. However, such programs should be confined to the known
and knowable. The court's almost casual assumption that the price advertising
it authorizes can be policed effectively by medicine or the bar reflects a striking
underappreciation of the nature and magnitude of the disciplinary problem.

The first to respond to this new climate of opinion signaled by the FTC
and the *Bates* decision was the New York State Board of Regents.[9] On July 28,
1977, they voted unanimously to permit physicians, dentists, and other professionals to advertise not only their services but also their prices in newspapers
and magazines. Regent Emlyn Griffith described the action as allowing "fac-
tually accurate and dignified advertising." Both the Supreme Court and the
New York Regents barred price advertising from radio and television because
"the possibility of abuse seemed to be greater in the electronic media than in
the printed media."

As one reviews the current scene, certain facts do seem to stand out. It is
becoming increasingly difficult for members of the general public to obtain
accurate information concerning the training, hospital affiliations, and practice
profiles of the physicians in their community. The most readily available
information comes not from medical directories found on library shelves but

from articles in the lay periodicals and the often incomplete physician directories assembled by consumer groups. The profession as a whole has failed to take a vigorous action to meet this public need even though it would appear incumbent on them to do so.

There seems to be a strong case for moving ahead with the preparation of medical directories which would include such information as e physician's name, address, year of graduation, medical school, postgraduate training, board certification and recertification, type and limitations of practice, membership in national medical organizations where admission is based on qualifications, hospital affiliations, and medical school affiliations. However, there is also a strong case against publishing this information in newspapers, magazines, and especially over the electronic media. The directories might be physician—and consumer—sponsored and approved by respected community organizations to give them greater credibility. The listing of fees should be approached with considerable caution and strict guidelines or standards established that would make a misinterpretation virtually impossible.

The state and national medical organizations should continue to search out misleading advertising that would exploit patients and lower the quality of medical care. It is necessary that they seek public support in their efforts to maintain rigid professional standards. There has never been a time when it was more important to have an informed public who will share medicine's concerns and its efforts in maintaining a high quality of care at the lowest possible cost.

NOTES

1. Sehnert, Keith, M.D., and Eisenberg, Howard, "How to Rate Your Doctor," *Ladies Home Journal*, October 1975.

2. Bacialli, Susan, "How to Choose a Family Doctor and Get the Best," *Good Housekeeping*, August 1976.

3. "The Doctors Guide," Medical Section, *Newsweek*, November 18, 1974.

4. "How to Develop a Local Directory of Doctors," *Consumer Reports*, vol. 39 September 1974.

5. Denenberg, Herbert S., "Citizens Bill of Hospital Rights," Pennsylvania Insurance Department, Harrisburg, Pennsylvania, April 1973, Denenberg, Herbert S., and Shapp, Milton, J., "Shoppers Guide to Hospitals in the Philadelphia Area," Pennsylvania Insurance Department, Harrisburg, Penn.., —— —— , "A Shoppers Guide to Dentistry," Pensylvania Insurance Department, Harrisburg, Pennsylvania, February 1973. —— , "A Shoppers Guide to Health Insurance," Pennsylvania Insurance Department, Harrisburg, Pennsylvania, December 1973., Denenberg, Herbert S., "The Shoppers Guide to Surgery," Pennsylvania Insurance Department, Harrisburg, Pennsylvania.

6. Schwartz, Dr. Leroy L.: "The Princeton Survey Relating to Physician's Directories," (personal communication).

7. Sammons, James H., M.D., "The AMA and Two Medical Societies Go To Trial," *AMA Newsletter*, vol. 9, no. 31, September 2, 1977.

8. Supreme Court Decision no. 76-316, *United States Law Week*, June 28, 1977.

9. Meislin, Richard J., "New York Regents Vote to Allow Doctors and Dentists to Advertise," *New York Times*, Friday, July 29, 1977.

Going Public on Health Care Reform

H. Cranston Lawton

10

    The publication in August of AEtna Life & Casualty's first advertisement about the need to contain health care costs may have seemed like a thunderbolt from the blue. In reality, it reflected several years of concern about the economic, legal, and social trends forcing the cost of a number of types of insurance toward unaffordable levels. Further, the advertisements are but the most visible part of a larger communications program directed to opinion leaders, policymakers, claimants, and policyholders.

    The decision to go public was based on several assumptions. We assume, first, that the health care cost problem will be solved—either by the health care system itself or from outside. Also, we believe that an essentially private system working in partnership with government is inherently superior to a bureaucratic system—in terms of both quality and cost. Further, it seems to us that all elements of the system are contributing to runaway costs and all elements share responsibility for bringing them under control. Finally, we believe that the consumer will ultimately determine the shape of the health care system and that he is basically fair and honest, but he must become better informed on the issues.

Opinion research shows that a large majority of the public believes the problem of health care costs has reached crisis proportions.[1] Between the end of 1975 and the middle of 1977, the percentage of people who were substantially or very concerned about costs rose from 84 to 92 percent. To deal with the problem, 69 percent favored federal or state control of hospital charges and doctor fees, and 33 percent favored federal takeover of private health insurance (up from 25 percent at the end of 1975). This suggests that unless we who are part of the system work cooperatively to contain costs, the public will expect government to act on its behalf.

One effect of health insurance is to insulate nearly every other element of the system from the economic consequences of its decisions. Lacking external economic restraints, the system also lacks the ability of self-correction through cost-benefit analysis. And benefit design and claim cost control programs give insurers only limited leverage on market forces that conspire to raise prices. It is vital for the public to understand the issues and to act in its own best interests. This is what AEtna is trying to promote through its communications program.

As recently as the spring of 1977, AEtna was communicating almost entirely within the industry and to lawmakers and policymakers. But that summer we took the issues to the public, using magazines and newspapers to reach opinion leaders, policymakers, and corporate executives. The advertisements each deal with one facet of the cost problem with as much balance as possible within the confines of a readable commercial message. AEtna advertisements employ provocative illustrations and headlines, backed up with candid language and documented statements. In anticipation of the interest that might be stimulated by the advertisements, we have prepared press backgrounders—papers that document the statements made in the advertisement and place them in a broader perspective for news writers. In total, this effort will present a comprehensive picture of the problem and alternative ways of solving it.

The response has been surprising because favorable and unfavorable comments have been about evenly split, and irritated readers are usually much more inclined to write. With one exception, all the adverse letters came from health care professionals, who complained of scapegoating. Presumably, the campaign will answer that understandable reaction as it unfolds.

In addition to the national advertising, AEtna will publish statewide messages to help develop informed local constituencies for health care cost containment, as legislatures consider programs for improving the distribution and financing of care. Also, AEtna's chairman, John H. Filer, has written to the chief executives of policyholder companies and of other leading corporations, a total of about 1,000 businessmen. The letter outlines the dimensions of the problem, suggests solutions, and invites support of federal and state legislation that would slow the rise of costs without impairing the quality of care. In addition, AEtna is enclosing messages with many of the 16 million claim payments made each year to the employees of policyholders. AEtna is also developing short articles about medical expense benefits to be distributed to the editors of employee publications.

One objective of this whole communications program is to help develop a better informed public and to define the systemic character of the health care cost problem. A second objective is to help create a climate that will make it possible to build on existing institutions to moderate costs while improving the distribution and enhancing the quality of care. There is no greater threat to quality than costs rising so fast that the middle-income group is made medically indigent, and there is no more tempting audience for a demagogue than a large population group that feels it is losing a basic right. Through its public issue advertising campaign and the communication program supporting it, AEtna believes it is helping to meet its responsibility to its customers and to society as a whole.

NOTE
1. *The Cambridge Report*, second quarter 1977.

Hospitals Face a Marketing Future

Donald R. Giller

11

Professors of marketing are prone to employ Ralph Waldo Emerson's classic adage in introducing their courses: "If a man . . . make a better mousetrap . . . the world will beat a path to his door!" These instructors cite Emerson not to agree but to disagree: it is not true that a good product necessarily means success in business. Without proper marketing, the professors say, the path to the Better Mousetrap Corporation will quickly become hidden in underbrush.

Marketing—those activities within an organization that serve to match the organization's production of goods and services with consumers' needs and wants—has always found ready justification in a loosely controlled society marked by an economy of plenty. Such a society has traditionally had competing interests in the business of building mousetraps, and consumers have been free to assume that the particular mousetrap they were buying was the best. In case of a mistake, a second purchase could easily be handled.

As we enter a period in which hospitals for the first time are beginning to apply the marketing process—or at least marketing-oriented thought—to their services, it is striking that the principal stimulus to this trend is a tightly controlled economy of scarcity. Confronted with regulation at every turn, subjected to society's demand that costs be moderated, hospitals—which seemingly were unneedful of marketing in a society of plenty—now appear desperate to apply its methods in their search for a healthy bottom line—or, indeed, survival.

Although I emphasize the difficulties that may lie ahead, I am convinced that the adaptation of marketing techniques to hospital needs is a timely, proper, and most probably enhancing trend. I welcome it. Nevertheless, it is important for those of us associated with hospitals to walk into the future with eyes open, and to recognize that we should add Problems and Pitfalls to the traditional "Four Ps" of marketing: Product, Price, Place, and Promotion.

The Quick Fix: Emphasizing Beds, Not Services

Hospitals bring to the world of marketing a heavy load of traditions, assumptions, and habits. Although current and proposed reimbursement practices mean that hospital revenues no longer hinge so directly on percentage of beds occupied, the hospital administrator new to marketing will be inclined to assume that a quick emphasis on an isolated marketing task—promotion, for example—will fill beds and solve problems.

Problem: Emphasis on the promotional part of marketing alone may net the patients necessary to fill the beds, but in the long term, as PSROs and other utilization review mechanism effectively tighten their standards, the quick-fix solution will become less tenable, if it can be carried out at all. By that time, we may expect hosptial marketing practices will themselves have developed greater sophistication.

The March of Progress: Research on the Decline?

Again looking at the short term and in concert with federal research priorities, academic medical centers in particular will attempt to quicken the pace at which advances from clinical and basic research are put into medical practice. This emphasis on clinical application will lead to a diminution of funding of—and institutional interest in—the kinds of basic and clinical research that earlier made today's applications possible.

Problem: The profit-oriented industries demonstrate that research and development play a dominant role in continuity of profit levels; but R&D tend to suffer in times of economic downturn, such as the hospital industry is experiencing today. The next few years will probably prove difficult ones for research. After a settling-out period, however, emphasis on R&D will return to sufficient levels.

Market Research: Will the Truth Out?

One of the first steps in organizing a marketing function is defining where one is starting from. The hospital must collate a body of facts that fully describe its patients, its physicians, and its services. This must precede any attempt to assess what further services and amenities the hospital can offer as its part of a successful exchange relationship.

Problem: The hospital may not like what it learns about itself—that its patients are less well off than supposed, that it serves less of a tertiary care need than imagined, and so on—and it may respond by blaming the data collector or interpreter, challenging the accuracy of the data themselves, or ignoring them. Again, this kind of behavior will prove to be a passing aberration, if only because sound futures need to be built upon more solid foundations than fantasy permits.

Doctors and Hospitals: Friends or Foes?

The very great majority of hospitals have traditionally acted less as coherent institutions than as groups of medical fiefdoms. Most often, the institution has found it advantageous to cede or subvert its own objectives to those of the medical department heads.

Problem: The future will require hospitals to assert their institutional prerogatives as never before, with short-term losses to those department heads who have become used to having their needs and desires accepted as the institution's own. A true market system, in which there is a mutuality of exchange, will ultimately prove to be the only kind of system that can flourish in the future. Creative service chiefs will work to have their own goals accepted as genuine institutional goals; those chiefs who fail to meet this test will fall by the wayside.

"Demarketing": What of the Patients?

Marketing in the hospital context is most often considered a way of planning new services. It is sometimes forgotten that the marketing function should also discover what services in the current repertoire are counterproductive of fiscal health.

Problem: It is presumably within a hospital's rights to close out a service, but what of its obligation to direct the patients (and their physicians) using the service in question to alternatives? Unless the hospital arranges, say, appropriate primary care for "inappropriate" emergency room patients, it may suffer a loss of community goodwill that will transfer to other of the hospital's programs. The point is that hospitals need to spend as much creative time in scaling down programs as in establishing new ones.

Will Public Concerns Hasten Examination of "Track Records"?

As a hospital begins to accumulate data about itself preliminary to a marketing program, it is likely that the data will also describe community health needs in general and services offered by other institutions and agencies.

Problem: Given the current public concern about hospital costs, might there arise demands that these data be made a matter of public record? It is likely that the data will be very valuable to health systems agencies (HSAs), which, despite their mandate to coordinate regional health planning, lack the mandate to learn as much about every hospital as each hospital can learn about itself. Continued filing of the limited information now required may satisfy certain agencies, but as knowledge about the wealth of marketing data spreads, there almost surely will be attempts to have hospitals share that wealth.

Marketing Here, Marketing There: Who's Evaluating Whom?

I have one final concern: how are we to evaluate all these marketing efforts: Hospital management must be careful to design an adequate system to control, as well as to plan and implement, the marketing function. It is important to the success of whatever system is devised to be able to know whether it works!

Problem: What measures can be used as an index of marketing effectiveness? Measurement of any one variable within a complex health care delivery system is a risky business, but certain possibilities come to mind.

Occupancy of specific clinical services

Number of procedures (e.g., laboratory, surgical)

Patient mix (demographic or disease variables)

Physician mix (geographic or specialty variables)

Fund-raising impact (particularly for marketing programs directed toward development)

Climate among opinion leaders, legislators, regulators, bureaucrats (important in marketing programs to effect favorable certificate-of-need decisions, for example)

I foresee the ultimate success of hospital marketing programs as—in a sense, at least—antithetical to the mission of HSAs. If hospitals, through successful marketing, are effectively controlling the health care system, what role will there be for HSAs? Such an outcome would further strain the already troubled HSA-hospital relationship.

Eyeglasses: The Public's Right to Know

Robert D. Reinecke

12

Our country's yearly public expenditures on eyeglasses, including sunglasses, is about $4.5 billion.[1] But—while spending all this money, how much do consumers actually know about the true cost and quality of eyeglasses?

Sources of Glasses

Consumers may obtain glasses in various ways. Some visit an ophthalmologist, an M.D. who specializes in medical and surgical eye care, who writes a prescription to be filled by an optician. Alternatively, the consumer may visit an optometrist, who is not an M.D. but who is trained in refraction techniques. The optometrist can prescribe spectacles and typically orders them from an optical supply house and fits them to the patient him or herself. Or, the consumer may visit one of the high-volume optical companies, who typically employ both opticians and optometrists, or, in some states, a department store may display spectacles over the counter (OTC). The person selects the strength lenses he wishes and leaves with the eyeglasses.

Some firms supply safety glasses, usually ordered directly from a large optical supply house, if an employee has a prescription from his optometrist or ophthalmologist. In other firms, a contract entitles employees and dependents to eye examinations and a certain number of eyeglasses per year. Often, groups of either ophthalmologists or optometrists are under contract to the company to serve its employees.

Four Myths in Buying Glasses

The average American logically expects that higher cost means better quality, but this turns out not to be the case for glasses. The cost of spectacles from an ophthalmologist and optician is about the same as from an optometrist, but both are higher than OTC commercial sources. No rigorous studies have been done to compare relative costs and benefits. However, spectacles bought over the counter meet higher standards than those specifically ground for patients on prescription.

Further, most patients believe that only one quality lens will satisfy their need, especially for higher powered lenses. Yet, there is a spectrum of prices available to the optician or the optometrist, but not usually made available to the patient.

Third, the public has been led to believe that different lenses placed before the eye will, in some way, affect the health of the eye, even though few would even consider that the quality of glass in a window or automobile windshield would affect the eye. The fact that only in a few isolated cases will the wrong lens have any adverse effect on the eye, and these are cases where the patient would be seeing an ophthalmologist frequently anyway and the error would be quickly detected.

The public has also been misled concerning the amount of light necessary for comfortable reading. The eye is capable of adapting so effectively to extremes of illumination that tinted lenses are rarely called for. If brightness is so great that it causes discomfort, then sunglasses that absorb significant amounts of light are appropriate.

Sunglasses and Reading Glasses

Most "sunglasses" are tinted only for cosmetic appeal: the tint is not of sufficient density to effectively filter bright light. The federal Food and Drug Administration's Committee for Ophthalmic Devices felt strongly that the light-transmission characteristics of sunglasses should be indicated and made suggestions to the sunglass industry about appropriate labeling. The industry indicated that it would probably not comply. The industry has noted that the lenses in a $10 pair of sunglasses are usually identical to those in a $70 pair, with price differential due to the frame.

The committee has heard testimony regarding the implied dangers of

OTC reading glasses, but no dangers were discovered. If such glasses were labeled with the dioptric power of the lenses, the consumer who knows the strength lens he needs could easily select appropriate glasses. The laws responsible in many states for prohibiting the sale of reading glasses OTC and for this bit of disguise in labeling are traceable to the vested interests of opticians and optometrists. These groups have used the tenuous argument that prohibiting OTC glasses forces consumers to have an eye examination, where, if disease is present, it will be detected and blindness prevented. However, the consumer has no assurance that an eye examination, especially from a non-M.D., will detect an eye disease in its early stages.

Arguments were also made before the committee that the consumer should be protected from the poor quality lenses found in OTC eyeglasses. This clearly implied that the $7–10 eyeglasses were not only defective, but would, as a result of their defects, cause harm to the eyes. However, further testimony proved that the quality of the lenses in these inexpensive spectacles was superior to those commonly given upon prescription. And, as I have mentioned, glass placed before the eye cannot affect the health of that eye.

Ophthalmologists versus Optometrists

Any relationship between optometry and medicine is remote. Optometry developed in response to a public need for refractions and glasses for the healthy patient. If the consumer is concerned about eye disease, then an ophthalmologist should be consulted.

Ophthalmologists and optometrists have developed an adversary relationship as the training of optometrists has expanded. The two now compete to some extent for the same patients and for industrial contracts for employee eye care. Companies and unions are evaluating competing presentations only on a cost basis, but no studies are available that relate the costs to the benefits of receiving care from one or the other profession.

However, neither group can do the work alone. If all patients were to go to ophthalmologists, that group would become overloaded and the public would suffer. Similarly, it would not be in the best interest of the public to channel all patients through optometrists—patients will often complain that they are not offered the opportunity of being examined by the most competent specialist. As a solution, the two groups should work out a relationship that ensures cross-referral so that patients will receive medical care when needed. State and federal legislation is exacerbating competition between ophthalmology and optometry, but industry may be in a position to promote the logical and efficient use of both groups.

What Government and Industry Need to Do

Any restrictions on the prescription of spectacles and any law that limits a person's ability to shop for the best price should be eliminated. Optical goods, clearly marked with their optical power, should be made available to the

American public over the counter, and should not be tied in any way to an obligation to have an eye examination. "Fashion eyewear" should be distinguished from sunglasses in the labeling of tinted lenses.

The adversary relationship that has developed between ophthalmologists and optometrists will continue in the foreseeable future, a fact that industry must take into account. Decisions involving the two groups should ensure clear lines of referral between them and give patients a choice of the level of professional they see. If possible, the triage should be done either on the basis of automated data collection or be done by the person most trained in disease—the ophthalmologist.

NOTES

1. Gordon R. Trapnell, "The Impact of National Health Insurance on the Use and Spending for Sight Correction Services," Optical manufactures Association, Arlington, Va., January 1977; and Drug Topics, Medical Economics Co., Oradeal, N.J., June 16, 1977.

Editors' note: for a recent newspaper account of the Federal Trade Commission's unanimous approval, on May 24, 1978, of new rules permitting advertising of prices and other information about eyeglasses, contact lenses, and eye examinations, see Carole Shifrin "FTC Approves Advertising of Eyewear Prices, Exam Data." Washington Post (May 25, 1978): A13.

ERISA: An Opportunity for Better Communication of Employee Health Benefit Plans

Linda Kay Stokes

13

The Employee Retirement Income Security Act (ERISA)[1] established important new reporting and disclosure requirements for employee benefit plans, including health plans. Besides specifying the information that plan administrators must provide to employees, ERISA requires that it be presented in understandable language, not in legal or technical jargon.

In part because ERISA's disclosure requirements were designed to regulate pension plans, compliance by administrators of other kinds of benefit plans has been neither easy nor inexpensive. Yet health benefit plan adminstrators may be too hasty in condemning ERISA as yet another example of officious federal meddling; the act may offer business and labor an opportunity to take important steps against the rising cost of health benefits. ERISA-required communications can be used not just to explain health benefits, but also to help employees become informed consumers of health care, to promote employee health, and to make employees more cost-conscious in their use of health benefits.

Simple Health Benefit Descriptions

ERISA requires each employee benefit plan adminstrator to provide a "summary plan description" that accurately describes benefits, eligibility rules, and employee rights in simple language. However, for all their detail and complexity, ERISA regulations actually offer little guidance for communicating complex health benefits in a nontechnical way. Some suggestions for understandable descriptions are presented here.

The summary plan description should make liberal use of illustrations and cross-references to help readers locate information in the text. In addition, its attractiveness will play a big part in its readability. Cartoons can be used and the amount of white space on pages can be increased by using a large, 8½" × 11" format.

The summary description should pay special attention to problem areas peculiar to the plan. If, for example, an unusually large number of participants are using hospital emergency rooms for primary care, the description should not only make it clear that these services are not covered (if in fact they are not), but it should also explain why this coverage is not provided and tell participants how to select and use a primary care physician.

The description should not rely on the detailed schedules of benefits provided by the insurer. Although ERISA regulations currently allow schedules, they are, with few exceptions, difficult to understand. Some insurer opposition to rewriting its "tried-and-true insurance language" should be expected, since all insurance forms must be filed with state insurance departments and any change in existing wording necessitates filing the new form in each state where it is used. Yet if enough policyholders insist on readable benefit descriptions, insurers will have to revise their materials, as some are doing, to meet the demand. In the meantime it will require give-and-take sessions between plan administrators and insurance company lawyers to hammer out health insurance schedules people can understand.

Comprehensive examples should be used to show how the plan's various benefits work together to provide coverage for a common medical incident, leaving the reader with a realistic notion of what the plan covers and how much would be left for him to pay. (See exhibit 1 for a sample illustration for an appendectomy.)

A recent benefit description for participants in a pension fund was returned with the comment, "If my husband could understand this, he wouldn't be a truck driver." One way to make sure the summary plan description is "written in a manner calculated to be understood by the average plan participant" is to show a draft of it to several average participants, and to their spouses, and ask if they understand it.

Information on Health Promotion and Consumption

While ERISA specifies the information the summary plan description must contain, it does not prohibit the inclusion of other information, as long as it is not false, misleading, or written in complex or confusing language. In

Exhibit 1
How your benefits work together when you are hospitalized

John had sharp pains in his side and went to his doctor. The doctor thought John had appendicitis, and ordered some laboratory tests and x-rays to be sure. The tests showed that John did have appendicitis, and he entered the hospital for five days for an appendectomy. Below is a list of bills he received for his treatment showing what was covered by his Basic and Major Medical Coverage and how much was left for John to pay himself.

Item	Bill	Basic Benefit Paid	Benefit
Basic Benefits:			
Diagnostic laboratory and x-ray tests (outpatient)	$75	$60	Outpatient diagnostic x-ray and laboratory expense benefit
Surgery (appendectomy)	300	275	Surgical benefit
Hospital room and board, 5 days	400	350	Hospital room and board benefit
Bandages, medicine, laboratory tests (inpatient)	250	200	Miscellaneous hospital expense benefit
Doctor visits	200	0	None
Total	$1225	$885 (paid by Basic Benefits)	

Major Medical Benefits:		*Total Benefits:*	
Eligible expenses not paid by Basic Benefits	$340	Total Bills:	$1225
Deductible (paid by John)	−100	Plan Paid:	−1077
		Difference	
		(not covered)	$ 148
Difference (Major Medical covers 80%)	$240 ×80%		
John's Major Medical Benefits	$192		

addition to describing health benefits, then, the summary plan description may also contain information to help employees become better informed consumers of health care and to promote employee health. ERISA-required benefit descriptions could carry the kind of information employees need in order to choose among providers and benefit plan options. The summary descriptions and comprehensive examples for each plan offered should be standardized and comparable in order to enable employees to decide, for example, whether to join a health maintenance organization or be covered by a group health insurance plan.

What is actually needed is a comparative value scale or a health benefit plan grading system to help consumers make their choices. At least one state (Minnesota) has developed such a grading system as part of its catastrophic health insurance law,[2] but it is too general to be very useful for finding the best plan for the money. Several national health insurance proposals have called for health plan grading systems, but in the meantime, perhaps either the insurance industry or business, as a large purchaser of health care, could develop a system to help both collective and individual health care consumers compare the value of benefit plan alternatives.

The summary plan description could also provide information to help consumers use their health benefits and the health care system more prudently and effectively. It might include, for example, information about the importance of having a primary care physician and some tips on how to select one. Suggestions for dealing more effectively with a physician, including how to ask questions about diagnoses, treatments, and costs, might also help employees get more out of their encounters with providers.[3] A discussion of how to find help for nonmedical problems affecting health might discourage inappropriate use of health care resources for problems that are social, financial, or legal in nature. A few words on the purpose of health insurance, as well as on the purpose of each plan benefit, could help to promote realistic expectations and appropriate utilization of health benefits.

Another possible use of the summary plan description is to give employees information to promote better health, including information about pertinent occupational health hazards and sources of diagnosis and treatment. It could also contain a self-care medical guide with information on such common problems as colds, fevers, burns, cuts, diaper rash, colic, poison ivy, and so on.

Finding good materials may be troublesome for plan administrators who wish to include information to promote employees' health and to teach them how to use the health system more effectively. The insurance industry, which has begun to develop these materials, may be encouraged to continue its efforts by more requests from business for this kind of information. Government could also play a role by supporting the development of information to teach consumers about smart, appropriate utilization of the health care system. Or business itself could take on the task, perhaps by establishing a clearinghouse for sharing useful information.

Information on Rising Health Care Costs

In addition to a summary plan description, ERISA requires the plan administrator to provide employees yearly information about the financial status of each benefit plan in a "summary annual report." This report, which also must be written in layman's language, is supposed to give participants enough information about benefit plan finances to enable them to protect their interests if the plans appear to be financially unsound. Required yearly, the summary annual report could become an effective vehicle for demonstrating the problem of health care cost inflation and for encouraging employees to become more cost-conscious in using their health benefits. Current ERISA regulations, however, stand in the way.

Considering that the summary annual report is supposed to communicate complex financial information to laymen, the regulations specifying its content are curious. It is entirely possible by following the regulations to come up with a summary annual report with all the readability of federal income tax Form 1040. Most items that must be included come directly from the plan's annual report, and the regulations effectively discourage an employer from trying to present this complex financial information any other way. Any additional information must not in any way conflict with or detract from the required information, and it is not surprising that few have considered editing and explanation a risk worth taking.

Yet the summary annual report could provide employees with helpful and interesting information about the cost of health benefits. As a yearly report, it could demonstrate the dramatic increase in health costs and break down cost increases by benefit. In addition, annual reports for alternative benefit plans could give consumers useful financial information for making informed choices among them. Such reports could form the informational basis of innovative health plans that reward employees who choose cost-effective health benefit plans and use them wisely.[4]

The federal government needs to take another look at the ERISA regulations for summary annual reports. In the first place, it is not clear that the regulations have lived up to their intent of giving participants enough financial information about their plans to protect themselves against plan mismanagement. Second, they make an employer run uphill to give employees additional useful information.

Summary

ERISA is requiring employers to expend considerable time and money to provide employees with information about their health benefit plans. Since it appears that ERISA is here to stay, employers might as well try to get their money's worth from their compliance efforts. Through creative compliance with ERISA's reporting and disclosure requirements, employers have an opportunity to help employees become more informed consumers of health care, to promote better employee health, and to make employees become more cost conscious in their use of health benefits. While current regulations do not prevent employers from giving employees this kind of information, neither do they provide them any incentive to do so. The federal government needs to develop better regulations governing the provision of health benefit plan information to employees. In the meantime, perhaps business should take the lead by trying out new methods and materials for communicating health information to employees.

NOTES

1. P.L. 93-406.

2. Minn. Stat. 62 A.04.

3. See, for example, Keith W. Sehnert, *How to Be Your Own Doctor (Sometimes)* (New York: Grosset & Dunlap, 1975).

4. See, for example, "Do Groups Really Deliver More Bang for the Buck?" Interview with Paul M. Ellwood, Jr., M.D., *Group Practice* 26: 18–22 (May-June 1977).

HCHP Successes and Failures in Communicating Information to Its Publics

Robert S. Lurie and Robert L. Biblo

14

The Harvard Community Health Plan (HCHP) is a prepaid group practice-type HMO serving some 70,000 members in the greater Boston area. Medical services, including outpatient, mental health, and emergency care, are provided in two multispecialty health centers, and inpatient services are provided at affiliated hospitals nearby. The Plan is recognized as a sound, stable, and high quality medical care institution, but its existence has not always been this secure. When its first center opened in 1969, it had staff and facilities ready to serve 10,000 members, but only 88 had joined. In fact, it was sixteen more months before membership reached 10,000, and almost three more years after that before the HCHP started operating in the black.

The barriers to early success were lack of knowledge of the Plan on the part of prospective members and some outright hostility from other quarters. A key to overcoming these barriers has been HCHP's development of a multifaceted marketing program. From the problems and successes of the HCHP, we may venture to predict the likely barriers that group practice HMOs will face and some strategies for overcoming them.

HCHP and Marketing

Marketing is not merely trying to make a sale to a customer. Rather, it has been described as "a systematic, disciplined approach for taking a product or service to the marketplace,"[1] and it must address a wide variety of publics. Health care marketing has been divided into four component parts: product, price, place, and promotion.[2]

HCHP's product is both medical services and health insurance. This fact is important in understanding the HCHP market because an HMO competes with a potential member's current health providers and with his or her current insurance. To be selected, HCHP had to be judged superior on both counts. However, the Plan has had to face the confusion and hesitancy that often greets a new product in the marketplace.[3]

The price of HCHP membership vs. traditional insurance is confusing to prospective members because of the effect of employer contributions. As a hypothetical example, if the HCHP family premium is $70 per month and the traditional insurance premium is $65, this does not appear to be a major difference. However, if the employer pays $60 toward either option, then the remainder is either $10 or $5—a 100 percent difference to the employee. Employees are not often aware of the considerable out-of-pocket savings that may result from an HMO's broader benefit package compared with traditional insurance plans, and in any case, a comparison of the total costs of the two options can be very complex.[4]

Place was a critical decision for HCHP because studies have shown that accessibility is a key determinant in the choice of a health care provider[5,6,7]. The first center's location was chosen because it is central to Boston, to the neighboring cities and towns and close to the affiliated hospitals. It can be reached easily by public transportation or by car. In addition, the physical plant is modern and colorful, a far cry from the traditional "clinic" image.

With a product that is new and complex, promotion is critical to marketing success. Yet this has generally been ignored in the short history of HMOs' evolution. HCHP, like many others, expected to find members easily,[8] and proceeded without sufficient market research and promotion, thus overprojecting enrollment. But marketing difficulties have been continually documented[9], and HMOs would be well advised to develop strategies to deal with these issues.

The Concept of Publics

A health care organization must promote itself to all its "publics," that is, to any group that "has an actual or a potential interest and/or impact on [the] organization"[10]. HCHP has many publics who influence its ability to achieve its marketing goals, including employees, employers, providers, and financiers, as well as external forces such as government and the media.

Employee publics include both current members and non members. The former are those whom the plan wants to satisfy and retain. In addition, the plan wants them to represent it positively to fellow employees, since talking with co-workers is a common occurence in choosing a health plan[11,12]. The group of non members includes some who have a physician and some who don't, as well as people new to the area. These three categories have different perspectives from which they will judge the plan and to which the plan must respond.

Promotion within the employer group public also has many dimensions. In order for the plan to be introduced and promoted successfully as a second health coverage option, the cooperation of many levels in the organization is required. The chief executive officer or the board typically chooses the plans to offer and the personnel director manages them, while the actual process of getting employees to sign up is often performed by a clerk. In addition, if an HMO wants to explain its plan to employees while on the job, the cooperation of supervisors as well as the employees themselves is needed.

The plan must also promote itself to its provider public, be they current staff, prospective staff, affiliated providers, or institutions. Issues such as financial incentives, terms and conditions of work, working environment, and peer recognition are all critical to current and prospective staff. Hospitals are concerned about aspects of payment and what effect this new supply of patients may have on the existing availability of beds. They are also concerned about the reaction of the existing medical staff in the hospital, as these physicians supply the hospitals with most of their patients and therefore their income source.

The HMO must also promote itself to potential financiers, who may be lenders, foundations, or government. Here promotion efforts must demonstrate the soundness of the management team, the quality of the provider team, the justification for membership projections, and the action plans for turning those projections into actual members.

Finally, but certainly not least in importance, there are a variety of external publics, including regulators, insurers, outside providers, and the media. Government has jurisdiction in various separate and overlapping ways over much of the plan's program and even has the ability to prevent operation.

The extent to which media coverage is favorable or unfavorable can support or negate other promotion efforts. The introduction of an HMO will disrupt the markets of current providers of its products, and it must expect some opposition and/or hostility from health care providers, insurers, and their associations.

An HMO must manage its promotion strategy vis-a-vis all its publics simultaneously. Also, it must understand and try to affect relationships of one public to another. For example, current members will be discussing the plan with potential members. Employers who offer HCHP may influence employers who do not. Government can be pressured by consumer groups, employer groups, and provider groups, as well as by the insurance and medical care industries. Or government may exert influence over some of them. What exists is the complex network of publics, dealing with the plan and with one another, that the plan must try to reach in its marketing efforts.

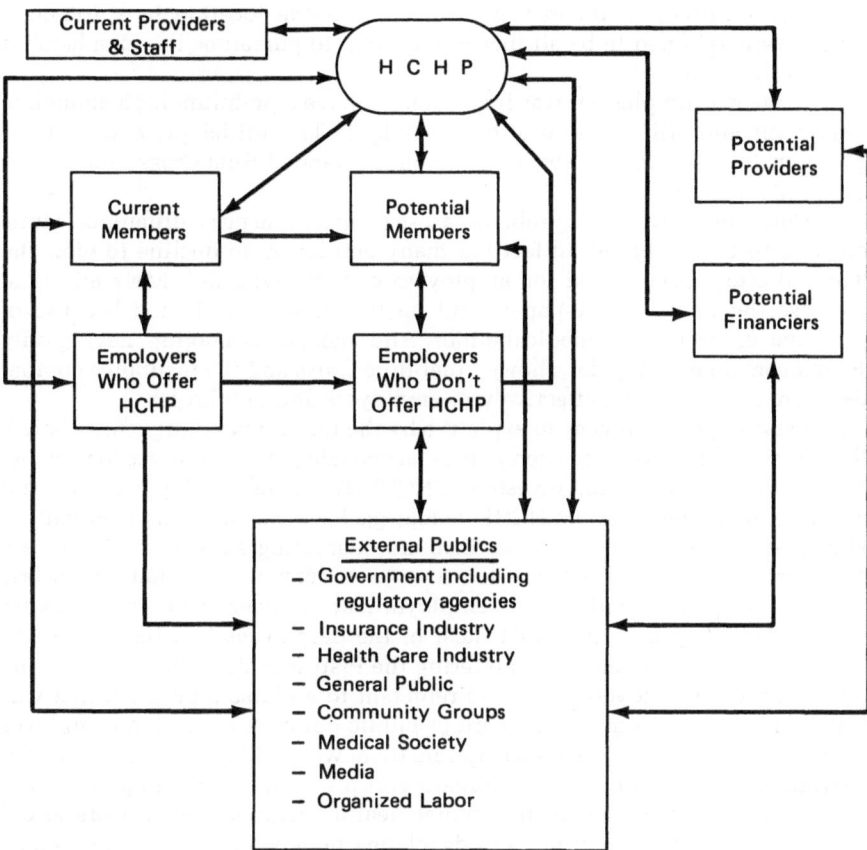

Figure 1
HCHP and its publics.

The First Four Years: Trying to Break Even

To open its first center, HCHP affiliated itself with four Harvard University teaching hospitals and recruited physicians who met the standards of Harvard Medical School and the teaching hospitals. Its product, it hoped, would be seen as at least equal in medical quality and broader in coverage than any fee-for-service alternative available in the Boston area. To overcome the likely hostility it would face, to make marketing easier, and to gain economies of scale from the insurers' administrative operations, HCHP entered into a first-of-its-kind partnership with Blue Cross and ten insurance companies to underwrite, market and provide certain other administrative services to the Plan while HCHP provided medical care. The insurers agreed to a membership quota or penalty system. This alliance, it appeared, would give additional credibility to the Plan and provide immediate entree to employers. This plus high-quality providers, broad benefits, and a central location in a first-class facility were assumed to be all that was needed to guarantee the membership needs of the Plan.

In the startup phase it was impossible to have a premium high enough to break even and still hope to attract members. The initial price was set at approximately $5 a month above the community-rated Blue Cross Blue Shield Master Medical premium.

However, a number of problems arose at once. The price difference, while intended to be negligible, in fact led many employers to decline to offer the Plan and often discouraged the employees of those who did. Early efforts to advertise the Plan in newspapers and on the radio were halted because of objections on grounds of medical ethics. And, most discouraging, having only 88 members on opening day showed that Blue Cross and the insurance companies were not marketing effectively to employers and employees.

In retrospect, it is easy to explain why the initial marketing efforts failed. Blue Cross and the insurance companies lacked adequate incentives to promote HCHP. They had no capital invested in HCHP; the penalties if quotas were not met were negligible; and the HCHP benefit package was in direct competition with their own package. Also, the insurers' marketing staff, with HCHP as a minor product line, did not take the time to understand the plan, much less explain it properly. Similarly, the employer had no incentive to offer another option when they perceived that most of the employees had insurance and access to medical care and when offering the Plan was an additional administrative burden. Employers were also reluctant to endorse a program that was controversial and had no track record or public policy support. If an employer was looking for a health insurance option, there were still many questions to be answered about the concept of a prepaid group practice and the operations of HCHP. Being accustomed to traditional health insurance, employers asked many questions about waiting periods, claims review, cost control programs, and conversion to nongroup insurance. Only after taking the time to ask these questions and listen to answers did employers begin to lower their resistance.

In order to avoid going bankrupt just a few months after opening its doors, the Plan had to initiate a two-pronged marketing effort. First, HCHP strengthened its contractual agreement with Bue Cross. Staff from Blue Cross were to be assigned full-time to selling the Plan and committed to achieving sizable monthly and cumulative membership quotas. In the event of a membership shortfall, Blue Cross would pay HCHP for the Plan's fixed costs. Second, HCHP hired its own staff to market the Plan to all employer groups where the ten insurance companies had a relationship.

The new marketing staffs lacked experience in marketing an HMO and knew very little about health care delivery in general and HMOs in particular. They certainly did not possess the detailed knowledge required to answer the questions raised by employers and employees. HCHP therefore put its own and Blue Cross's teams through intensive training by the Plan's management and its medical staff. Afterward, HCHP initiated a desperation marketing effort which proved to be effective.

The gross overstaffing of the Plan at this time, while a financial disaster, was turned to a marketing advantage. Prospective members were encouraged to visit the center and talk with Plan providers about the program during "get acquainted" sessions. Once enrolled, new members found that appointments were readily available and visits with the physicians and nurses were leisurely. However, as the Plan grew and its providers began to have a typical workload, some of the early members perceived a drop in the level of service. It was difficult for them to see that this was only a return to normalcy, not a program falling apart.

Another early marketing technique was to stress preventive care, and members were encouraged by marketing staffs to come in for an initial physical exam. Again, as the Plan grew and physicians were not as readily available for these routine physicals, members were upset. These experiences show that it is risky for a plan either to oversell itself or to offer its members a level of service that it cannot maintain over the long run.

Just as HCHP began to solve some of its membership difficulties, the problem of getting and keeping physicians began to emerge. Qualified physicians were not always available in every specialty at exactly the time staff were needed. Also, HCHP's financial woes were becoming known to the general medical community and this made it difficult for the Plan to attract new physicians as it grew. Fortunately, the Plan was able to take advantage of support from its other publics. Grants and loans totalling $800,000 were received, serving to solidify the Plan's financial position and to show prospective providers that the foundation and financial communities considered it viable. In addition, the Plan received continued endorsement from Harvard Medical School.

Of all the external publics, the ones most hostile to the Plan were selected district medical societies. After a few years, however, this opposition quieted. Presumably the Plan's location in downtown Boston represented little threat to fee-for-service physicians located mostly in the suburbs.

The Plan did try to gain support from labor unions, consumer groups, and local professional associations. Even when these efforts met with success, the Plan learned that the endorsements had little impact in recruiting members or even getting employers to offer the Plan. As a result, HCHP followed, with success, the strategy of making a breakthrough with one or two employers in a particular field and then using them to help gain entree to others. This approach was particularly effective among colleges and universities and among law offices. The Plan's promotion strategy in subsequent years has also focused on the annual reenrollments from employer groups. Early members had a chance to try out the Plan and give their stamp of approval or disapproval to their fellow employees. From many such groups came growth at the time of reenrollment, representing as much as a doubling of the membership from an employer.

As a result of all these efforts, 1971 and early 1972 brought continual, almost frenetic growth. The Plan quadrupled its membership, reaching 30,500 members in July 1972, while the number of participating employers jumped from less than 200 to over 800. The latter part of 1972 and most of 1973 was a period of recovery and adjustment, as illustrated in figure 2. At this time the Plan discovered that its membership turnover exceeded 25 percent per year. However, surveys indicated that this turnover was not explained by members'

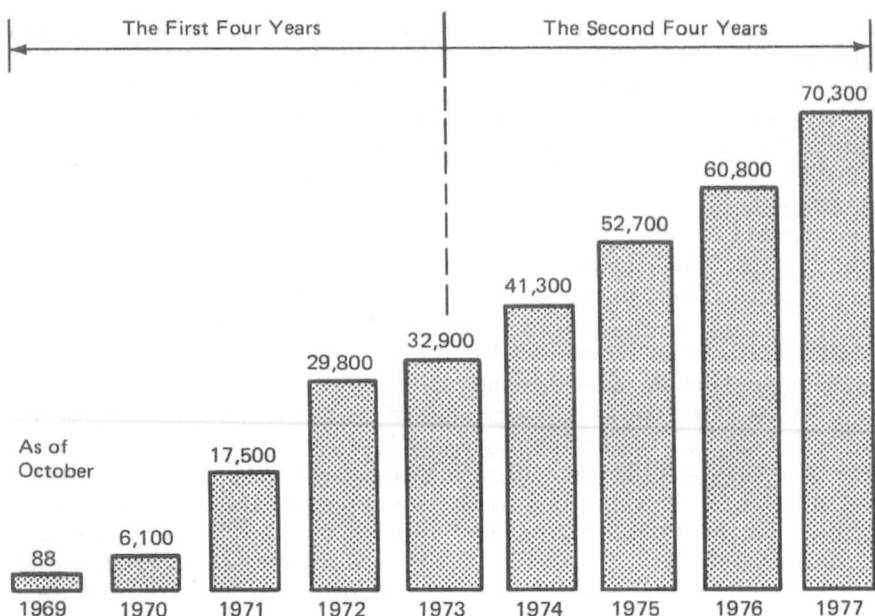

Figure 2
HCHP membership history, 1969–1977.

dissatisfaction. Instead, almost 85 percent of it was due to members' moving out of the service area or changing to an employer who did not offer the Plan. Therefore, HCHP negotiated a new quota agreement with Blue Cross. The new target was a "net quota," that is, the number of members that Blue Cross would enroll above and beyond replacing those who terminated.

Also during this period many of the Blue Cross marketing staff who had gone through the Plan's training program and had worked so closely with Plan marketing staff to achieve its rapid growth were promoted or reassigned. Their replacements never achieved the same understanding of or commitment to the Plan, and Blue Cross also demanded that HCHP no longer have contact with Blue Cross accounts for either enrollment or servicing. Not surprisingly, the new staff never enjoyed the successes of their predecessors.

The Second Four Years: Solidifying the Plan

During 1973 there were many significant events that altered the relation-ship of the Plan with its publics. First, the Plan opened a second health center in Cambridge, bringing opposition from some Cambridge fee-for-service physi-cians. A group of them opposed the Plan's getting a certificate of need, but support from Cambridge Plan members helped to neutralize this opposition.

A second important milestone occurred during this period when HCHP had its first three months of financial operations in the black. This strengthened its credibility with the financial community, but it was achieved only after a substantial premium increase. The Plan could no longer subsidize operating losses through grants and loans, but had to achieve self-sufficiency. As expected, the new premium impeded growth, but HCHP had already anticipated this in its budgetary planning.

At the end of 1973 came the passage of the HMO Act, endorsing and promoting the growth of HMOs. After passage of new HMO amendments in 1976, HCHP sought and obtained federal qualification. The major advantage of the HMO Act was the dual-choice requirement; however, it is important to remember that merely having the plan offered does not guarantee new membership. It continues to be necessary for an HMO to manage carefully its relationship with its employer and employee publics.

HCHP was beginning a new era in dealing with its publics. Gradually, it improved its premium position relative to the competition. Between 1974 and 1977, the HCHP family premium went up by approximately 36 percent, while the Blue Cross Master Medical community-rated family premium went up by 94 percent (see figure 3).

HCHP also recognized that employers were finally becoming extremely concerned about the cost of health insurance premiums. In those groups where the HCHP premium was less than the premium for traditional insurance and the employer was contributing most or all of the cost, the Plan developed a strategy of price marketing to the employer—representing itself as a way to save money.

In the summer of 1974 HCHP was offered, for the first time, to state employees. Because of the large potential market there, the HCHP marketing staff devoted much of its energy to getting new members from this group. As a result of a broader benefit package, a favorable premium differential ($35 per month per family contract in 1977), and the option of two health centers, membership by state employees accounted for almost one-third of the Plan's growth from 1973 to 1977.

Recent Developments and Prospects for the Future

During the latter part of its second four years HCHP became increasingly concerned about its dependence on Blue Cross's ability and desire to meet HCHP's marketing objectives. The Plan also concluded that Blue Cross's charge for marketing and certain administrative services was at least $1 million per year more than it would take the plan to perform the same services itself. The economies of scale in the Blue Cross relationship had not materialized.

Just as the Plan was questioning this relationship, the Commonwealth of Massachusetts became very supportive. The governor issued a white paper in support of HMO development[13], and the legislature made it legal for HMOs to operate independently of a relationship with the insurance industry. As a

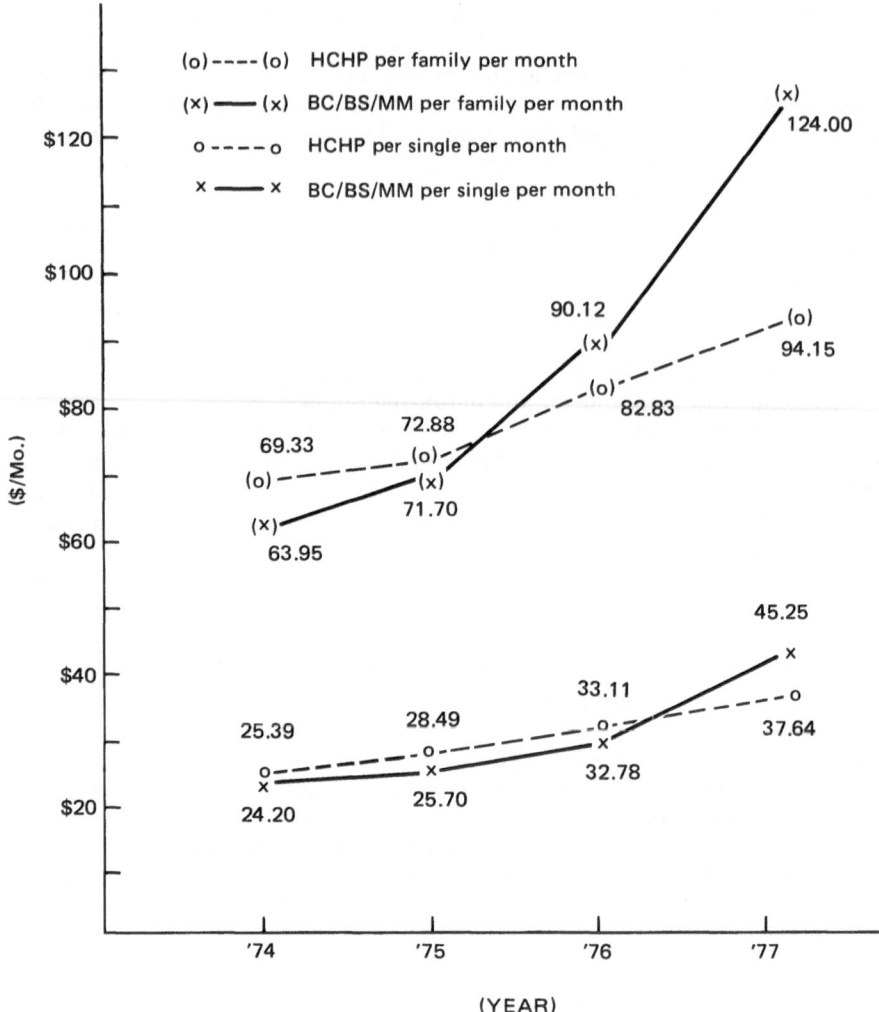

Figure 3
Monthly premium rates for family and single subscriber units: HCHP and Mass.
Blue Cross, Blue Shield, Master Medical (community-rated groups), 1974–1977.

result, in 1977 the Plan phased out its relationships with Blue Cross and the insurance companies and now contracts directly with all employer groups.

In December 1976 the Plan issued a long-range planning report that calls for, among other things, growth up to 175,000 members by 1982. As existing centers are reaching capacity, it is clear that the plan must open additional centers to achieve this objective. However, in developing its marketing strategy over the next five years, HCHP can look to a very different relationship with its publics than it had in the past.

The Future: Positive Influences

The Plan is no longer a new and risky venture; it is firmly established as a financially viable health care system with premiums equal to or less than most competitive community-rated insurance plans. It has the federal endorsement that comes from being a qualified HMO and the legal right to be offered by employers as one option. And now that HCHP deals directly with all employer groups, it has greater control over account relationships, communication of information, and promotion of enrollment. The Plan no longer has to scurry frantically after new members; instead, it can plan its marketing strategies carefully.

Attracting providers is also less of a problem than it was in the early years. The Plan is now a secure place to work and has developed some prestige in medical circles.

HCHP has the additional advantage that resistance to advertising is breaking down. Advertising enables an HMO to communicate with a broad population who cannot be contacted by its small marketing staff, including the employees of certain large accounts, such as federal and state employees who may work in a variety of locations. Advertising enables the HMO to state its case in the way it deems appropriate; it does not depend solely on the interest, accuracy, and biases of an individual reporter. Used for purposes of consumer education about premiums, hours of service, location of facilities, description of benefit packages, explanation of emergency service, and so on, advertising can provide another mechanism to assist consumers in making intelligent choices.

The advertising issues that will shortly confront HMOs, as competition grows in the health care system, are more complex. Should the HMO begin to deal with quality issues? Why is it possible to provide more benefits at a lower premium than other providers? How significant are the limitations of an HMO system, such as a closed panel of providers? Should an HMO risk the criticism that will surely come after it raises these issues in the form of advertising? Because the public has a right to documented information and because injecting competition is of value in the health care field, the decision should be that raising these questions is an obligation.

The Future: Possible Obstacles

Changes relative to other publics cloud the future somewhat. Because of its independence from Blue Cross and the insurance industry, HCHP for the first time is in open competition with them. In response to its growth, HCHP can anticipate that insurance companies either will offer increased benefit packages or attempt to keep their premiums down by increased deductibles and copayments. Under pressures from government regulation and competition, the traditional system is likely to respond with lower hospital utilization, cutting into a prepaid group practice's major competitive edge[13]. Also, because any future markets that HCHP would tap are predominantly in the suburban areas, resistance from fee-for-service physicians may resurface. It is likely that individual practice HMOs (IPAs) will be formed.

Though the present governor is supportive of HMOs, it is possible that state government will be an obstacle in the future. HCHP is dependent on the Department of Public Health to approve, under the certificate of need program, any plans to open new ambulatory care centers. The Division of Insurance, in trying to develop a proper mechanism for regulating this new HMO movement, could adopt a stringent, burdensome, or even inappropriate approach. Also, it is uncertain how any state (or federal) health insurance program might affect the plan.

HCHP must also contend with hospitals in the future. Hospital affiliation requires dealing with each of a hospital's major centers of power: its management, its board of trustees, and its fee-for-service physicians. When HCHP first looked beyond the Harvard hospitals for affiliations, opposition was overwhelming. The threat to the hospital's existence was expressed in terms of lower bed utilization, less diagnostic testing, poor medicine, and so forth. In addition, there was the fear that somehow this unfamiliar entity would sink its fangs into a once proud hospital, dominate it, and change it.

Over the last year HCHP has seen some eroding of this solid hospital front. The more balanced publicity given to HMOs, the track record of HCHP in particular, and the favorable comments by HCHP members have created limited but significant changes. Some hospital boards of trustees, concerned with the severe inflation in the health care field, have perceived certain advantages in HMO relationships. Many administrators, caught between the regulatory crunch and a falling bed census, similarly see a value in an HMO affiliation.

Unfortunately, this is not the case with the hospital's fee-for-service staff. In fact, the strong support from HCHP's other publics may have created additional fears. There have been instances where a hospital's fee-for-service staff have voted unanimously against any affiliation with HCHP. Physician opposition arises from fear of loss of income through competition, fear of inadequate bed space for their own patients, and general hostility toward any concept that challenges the exclusiveness of fee-for-service practice. The HMO movement has generally not succeeded in winning over fee-for-service medical staffs. It is hard to say whether this is because of poor communication or whether, in fact, the HMO has communicated its message very well and that the fears of the fee-for-service world are well-founded. Any defense against this hostility will be most effective when it reaches large numbers of consumers and regulatory bodies.

Conclusion

One key to HCHP's meeting its future growth objectives will be for it to continue doing that which it has done well: providing satisfactory services and controlling costs. It is also important to develop expanded marketing strategies with each of its publics consistent with its new relations with them. HCHP may follow the example of other HMOs[14] by involving its medical and support staff more closely in its member relations program. It may also seek more input from members about improving the Plan.

Since the medical care, health insurance, and economic environments are changing, the Plan must continue to learn about these and other factors affecting choice of medical care programs and develop new promotion strategies in order to compete effectively. HCHP must also admit what it can and cannot do. It should welcome being evaluated against available alternatives. Finally, HCHP must simultaneously increase its financial strength and maintain its reputation for high-quality services. It is with balanced growth in all these areas that HCHP will be most likely to achieve its long-range plan.

NOTES

1. Nat N. Wexler, "What is Marketing?" *Hospitals: Journal of the American Hospital Association*, 51 (June 1, 1977).

2. Robin E. MacStravic, "Marketing Health Care Services: The Challenge of Primary Care," *Health Care Management Review* (Summer 1977):9–15.

3. Kenneth R. Davis, *Marketing Management* (Ronald Press, 1966).

4. Richard E. Weinerman, "Patients' Perceptions of Group Medical Care," *American Journal of Public Health*, (June 1964) 880–889.

5. Avedis Donabedian, "An Evaluation of Prepaid Group Practice," *Inquiry*, 6:3–25 (September 1969).

6. Klaus J. Roghmann, et al., "Who Chooses Prepaid Medical Care: Survey Results from Two Marketings of Three New Prepayment Plans," *Public Health Reports*, 90:516–527 (November–December 1975).

7. Richard Tessler and David Mechanic, "Factors Affecting the Choice between Prepaid Group Practice and Alternative Insurance Programs," Milbank Memorial Fund Quarterly, *Health and Society* (Summer 1973): 271–317.

8. Robert L. Biblo, *Marketing Pre-Paid Health Care Plans*, U.S. Department of Health, Education, and Welfare, 1972.

9. Robert M. Heyssel and Henry M. Seidel, "The Johns Hopkins Experience in Columbia, Maryland," *New England Journal of Medicine*, 295:1225–1231 (November 25, 1976).

10. Philip Kotler, *Marketing for Nonprofit Organizations* (Englewood Cliffs, N.J.: Prentice-Hall, 1975).

11. Charles A. Metzner and Rashid L. Bashshur, "Factors Associated with Choice of Health Care Plans," *Journal of Health and Social Behavior*, 8 (December, 1967); Roghmann, *op. cit.*

12. Claudia B. Galiher and Majorie A. Costa, "Consumer Acceptance of HMOs," *Public Health Reports*, 90:106–112 (March–April 1975).

13. Commonwealth of Massachusetts, "HMO Development Strategy for Massachusetts," 1976.

14. Lawrence Goldberg and Warren Greenberg, *The Health Maintenance Organization and Its Effects on Competition*, Federal Trade Commission, Bureau of Economics, 1977.

15. Health Insurance Plan of Greater New York, *This is How We Do It*, Pub. no. 115-9-67-5M.

Information Barriers to HMO Development

Kenneth J. Linde and George B. Strumpf

15

Mr. P. was confused. Mr. P had had Blue Cross Blue Shield health insurance since his employment began seven years ago, and in fact, this coverage was one of the reasons he had accepted his position with the company. A week ago, he received a letter from his employer stating that he must go to room 222 at 1:00 P.M. on October 13 to "hear a presentation on issues important to health care of himself and his family." After talking to fellow workers he found that only certain persons had received the letter and most were told to go to different rooms at different days and times. At home he discussed the letter with his wife but neither could divine the purpose of the meeting.

Mr. P arrived at the meeting early because he wanted to make sure that he

*A special note of thanks is given to John Lanigan, expert appointment, Division of Health Maintenance Organizations, whose work contributed to developing the marketing concepts that are needed to overcome barriers to HMO development.

missed nothing concerning so vital an issue. A young salesman, Mr. A, began to talk about a new health care plan that was being offered to all employees. It would mean giving up BC-BS coverage and joining something called the Midvale Health Plan, which, as far as Mr. P could discern, was one facility with full-time physicians that would provide almost all his health services either there or at Midvale Hospital.

When Mr. P asked who the physicians associated with the plan were, Mr. A replied, "The local medical society does not allow us to give out our list of physicians because this would constitute advertising of medical care," but he added that after joining the employee would be given a list of all primary care physicians and could choose one. Later, Mr. P learned that Midvale had two primary care physicians to choose from as well as access to various specialists and that more physicians would be employed as new enrollees joined. Mr. P liked the fact that all office visits would be covered but was unsure of going to one facility, being able to be admitted to only one hospital, and having to actually return his BC-BS card for this new, unknown organization. He was told he had three days to make up his mind. He and Mrs. P pondered about what he should do; it was difficult to assess and comprehend in such a short time.

Mr. P, three days later, decided that this new plan was too unclear to him and his wife. He decided to continue his BC-BS coverage and felt greatly relieved about his decision. His experience is an example of the informational barriers that impede HMO development.

Barriers to HMO Development

Reaction to HMOs has come from almost everywhere in the public and private sectors. Much of it reveals the confusion and skepticism that abound on this subject. It is known today that HMOs cost less than traditional delivery mechanism, but there exist some difficulties in relaying this to the employer and the employee. Obstacles can be found in marketing approaches, relations with the private sector, the lack of federal technical assistance, and the types of literature presented to the consumer.

Marketing Approaches

Nothing happens until somebody sells something. HMOs may decide to hire their own marketing staff or to work through brokers, Blue Cross, Blue Shield, a commercial insurer, and/or community groups. However, all these approaches have been plagued by problems. These arise from the newness of the HMO concept and its limited track record, industry's bias toward existing insurance programs, noncompetitive rate structures, and limited or absent financial support. Further difficulties may arise from inaccessible HMO facilities, limited physician participation, inexperienced marketing staff, the HMO's association with the federal government, and the lack of advertising.

One of the most important consequences for an HMO of all these barriers is revealed in unpublished data from the 1975 Health Interview Survey: over 70 percent of persons twenty years or over had never heard of a prepaid group practice (PGP). Of the 19.9 percent who answered that they had, only 4.3 percent could actually name an existing plan.[1] It is imperative that an HMO's sales representative be able to present a clear and concise benefit picture related to dollar expenditures and to answer any questions a potential participant might have. Employers will want to know what kind of health care is offered by the HMO, what services are included, how much must be paid by the employer, his employee, family members, and what the claims-handling mechanism is. Employees also may have questions—that is, if they even know about the plan. Too often marketing efforts are so oriented toward getting the approval of the union and the employer that no information is given to the employee, thus creating the ultimate unnecessary informational barrier.

The HMO's job in enrollment is not over when it signs new members, because the employee who has joined needs to be assured of quality care with as little "hassle" as possible. This makes it imperative that the proper service protocols be established to ensure that gains do not turn into losses.

Mandatory Dual Choice

The new mandatory dual choice offering should eventually remove many of these barriers. It is interesting to note that many qualified plans are not "leaning" on the dual choice rule as a threat to employers, but we believe that it has increased the number of participating employers. However, it should be remembered that mandatory dual choice is only for the employer and will not help to overcome any barriers associated with the employees. Many points of resistance to joining an HMO remain.

One of these is the "unbundling of benefits." When HMOs request dual choice, companies sometimes reply that they receive all their employee insurance—health care, accidental death and disability, life, and so on—through one insurer or broker and they do not wish to work with more than one for reasons of cost and time. Another source of problems is the Employee Retirement Income Secutity Act (ERISA). Employers sometimes state that HMOs are not included in their ERISA plans, and thus are reluctant to include them because of the extremely poor financial condition of many new HMOs. Companies often resist working with programs that are running in the red—that is, all federally qualified HMOs receiving loans.

At times there has been a problem of overselling that reflects poorly on all HMOs. Established broker or supplier relationships are also a problem as they are often difficult for new HMOs to compete with. In addition, subscriber contracts that require a percentage or a specific number of people to be enrolled in order to initiate a group plan may be set high enough to exclude HMOs de facto.

Finally, problems arise from such practices as cutting off hospital privileges to doctors who work part-time for an HMO or not referring patients to them. All these barriers persist despite the dual choice regulation and the federal certification of qualified HMOs.

Federal Educational Programs

An HEW recommendation dating from 1971 has been validated by recent experience.[2] This was that the expansion of HMOs be preceded by an effective effort to inform consumers about HMOs. Unfortunately, owing to resource limitations and the lack of clear statutory authority, no extensive federal education campaign has been possible. This, we feel, is one of the most significant problems in the federal HMO program. The government's concentration has been on developing new plans—numbers, if you will—because Congress, the administration, and others base success on how many HMOs there are, how many enrollees, and so on. But federal help with education is needed in all areas—for the staff of the HMO as well as for the community-at-large. Many HMO programs have reported that a great deal of opposition could have been avoided had there been a better education effort.

Relations with the Private Sector

There is growing evidence that a major, long-term influence on the growth of HMOs is the commitment of the private sector—unions and industry. As more of the private sector gains experience with HMOs, as HMOs maintain their cost containment statistics, and as traditional health care programs become increasingly expensive, there could be an increasing demand to have HMOs available to employees. But expansion will occur only if the private sector sees actual cost savings and an improvement in the delivery system. Meanwhile, there may be significant activity in the area of industry-sponsored health programs. In either case, industry is the key to the future direction of health care.

HMOs must find ways to develop credibility with the private sector so that a better relationship may be fostered. Some guidelines that can be used in the marketing program for this purpose are:

Established insurers have large support staffs, actuarial expertise, marketing statistics, and financial and managerial expertise, as well as financial reserves, all of which make for an easier paper transaction for the employer. To compete against this strong, established system, HMO representatives must be aggressive.

HMO representatives must be honest, explaining the disadvantages as well as the benefits and all program features to both employers and employees.

HMO representatives should sell only to employers whose program can be enhanced by the additional system.

Once arrangements with employers are closed, representatives should not "hang around" the corporation unless requested to sell the program. After sales, provide good service only when needed.

Update, on a continual basis, members benefit information and policy/procedural changes of the HMO.

Provide a mechanism for continuous employer and consumer relations.

HMOs have a limited but proven track record. As of the October 1977 quarter, the twenty-nine federally qualified HMO plans showed enrollment increases of 45,818 members or 18.4 percent. Annualized hospital days per 1,000 members for this quarter were 363 days for group practice models, down from 423 days during the previous quarter. Individual practice models showed 490 days compared with 443 days last quarter, and staff models, 439 days, compared with 369 days last quarter.[3]

Lack of Federal Technical Assistance

The Secretary of HEW should obtain additional staff especially with expertise in marketing, actuarial and financial management; issue all final regulations; and identify problems with state laws.[4]

This statement implies the numerous entry barriers that HMOs face in the health care market. Marketing expertise is perhaps the most crucial issue, but the above statement also indicates that the federal government itself is an entry barrier to the HMOs because of its lack of technical assistance. The undersecretary of health for the Department of Health, Education, and Welfare, Hale Champion, however, recently stated:

> I think HMOs have often been ill-served by the Department of which I am now Undersecretary, and the Secretary and I have agreed we are going to try to do a whole lot better in the future. All things won't happen right away. The disarray and debris left behind by people who didn't believe government could help solve problems or speed progress will take some time to clear away. Attitudes will have to change and so will aspirations. But if we rebuild mutual confidence in social progress, then we'll begin to actually make some again.[5]

Marketing Literature

A major requirement for the success of an HMO is the dissemination of accurate, comprehensive, and convincing material. It would be helpful to ensure that HMO representatives have the following available to take to small group meetings: sales brochures, rates, comparison sheets, perhaps a letter to the spouse if unable to attend, application (dual choice) card, and telephone number to call for any questions thought of after the presentation. It is suggested that all employees fill out an enrollment card to either continue their present coverage or join the new HMO plan. This will truly help to educate the employee as to the real meaning of dual choice.

Information that is developed for presentation to employees could consist of, for the total developmental and marketing effort, the following: "tickler"—for both employee and spouse, sales benefit package, how-to-use guide, and a comparison chart of HMO versus the most common BC-BS program (or other insurer). These four pieces of literature will help to provide clear information about the new health care plan.

Sales Tickler: This brief descriptive piece of literature is designed to arouse curiosity for additional information in the potential enrollee.

Sales Benefit Package: This may be used in the presentation sent to prospective members who request information about the plan.

How-to-Use Guide: This is a membership utilization brochure designed to assist the enrollee in learning procedures of the HMO. It covers such topics as using the program, making appointments, and grievance procedures.

Comparison Sheet: This is perhaps the most valuable piece of literature and could even be used for decision making by those who cannot attend the marketing presentations. It should be simple and easy to read.

The employee, employer and the HMO should always remember that Market Retention = Education and Service. The member must be aware of how to use the HMO; the staff of the HMO must be polite and helpful. The subscriber's experience during treatment at the HMO will help to determine the success of the plan. Well thought-out grievance procedures, newsletters, and other public relations will overcome even more barriers.

Since the majority of federally qualified HMOs have only recently marketed their product, little is known about the barriers to reaching the employee. Marketing approaches must identify potential consumers and their concerns and analyze the marketing procedures of traditional forms of health insurance. Through proper use of marketing procedures and literature, a more supportive posture by the federal government, and improved relations with the private sector, HMOs stand a strong chance of becoming a major factor in the health care delivery system.

The Potential of HMOs

Although the barriers to HMO development are many, it is important to recognize that HMO growth in recent years has been strong. From 1965 to 1975 there has been a continuous growth in HMOs, at the rate of approximately 15 percent a year.[6] A 1977 census shows 165 plans with 6,330,676 members. Sixty of the 165 are community-sponsored, 106 are group practice plans, and 50 are less than two years old.

While HMO growth has been endorsed by the administration and the Congress, the plans still have significant problems to face and still need support. Industry, consumers, government, and others must be vocal, organized, and persistent in their support of HMOs if the consumer is to have a meaningful choice of health care systems.

NOTES

1. Unpublished data, 1975, Health Interview Study, National Center for Health Statistics, Department of Health, Education, and Welfare.

2. Department of Health, Education, and Welfare, *Toward a Comprehensive Health Policy for the 1970s: A White Paper* (Washington, D.C.: Government Printing Office, 1971), pp. 31–32.

3. Division of Health Maintenance Organizations, DHEW Administrative material.

4. Report to the Congress, *Factors that Impede Progress in Implementing the Health Maintenance Organization Act of 1973*, Department of HEW, HRD 76–128, December 3, 1976, p. ii.

5. Hale Champion, Undersecretary of Health, Education, and Welfare, before the Group Health Association of America, Los Angeles, June 20, 1977.

6. Division of Health Maintenance Organizations. DHEW Administrative material.

Barriers to Promoting Prepaid Dental Programs

Joseph Boffa and Barry Rabner

16

    Though still lagging behind group medical insurance, group dental insurance has grown dramatically from 4 million people covered in 1967 to 34 million in 1975. An even more recent phenomenon is the prepaid group dental practice (PGP), found predominantly in the Midwest and West, and covering about 2 million people.

    The PGP has demonstrated a number of advantages. As an alternative to conventional insurance, with its deductibles and benefit limitations, maximums and copayments, costly claims processing, and so on, the PGP has been shown to decrease out-of-pocket expenses for the patient and administrative expenses dramatically. The advantages of a PGP to the provider derive from the protection capitation provides from seasonal cash flow fluctuations and short-term economic downturns. Finally, because the PGP managers know the size and demography of the population they serve, they can accurately and thoroughly plan to meet the needs of their patients.

    If dental PGPs are a good idea whose time has come, why have they lagged so far behind the growth of regular indemnity insurance? One would expect a system with all these advantages to gain wide acceptance; yet PGP plans represent less than 10 percent of the total dental prepayment market.

One barrier to growth is their need for management technology and highly sophisticated skills. For instance, if both prepaid and fee-for-service patients are seen in the same practice, there must be a management information system that can distinguish the time devoted to, and the income derived from, the two types of practice. Another barrier is that in some states guaranteeing a service for a fixed premium falls into the domain of insurance. Because insurance statutes frequently require substantial capitalization ($200,000 and up) and the maintenance of liquid reserves, group practices, even large ones, are discouraged from venturing into prepayment arrangements. Finally, a hurdle of major consequence has been a negative bias in the dental profession against group practice in general and capitation in particular.

In order for a PGP to flourish, two basic requirements must be met. First, services must be rendered on a contractual basis *solely* by members of the group or members of a network of solo practitioners. Second, the PGP must be free to develop marketing strategies both to penetrate the existing dental prepayment market and to attract persons now without coverage. This market is currently dominated by insurance companies and profession-sponsored insurance plans (such as Delta Dental).

Unfortunately, it is these two aspects of dental capitation that have encountered the most resistance from organized dentistry. Like physicians, dentists often object to closed panels on the ethical grounds that consumers cannot freely choose their practitioners. The American Dental Association in 1967 passed the following resolution: "[We are] opposed in principle to closed panel systems because of the essential limitation which this method of practice imposes on the patient. Closed panel practices must not be established except under special circumstances to meet the needs which cannot be met in any other way."[1] In 1971 a compromise resolution to allow dual choice options was submitted to the ADA but rejected.[2] What passed was a resolution calling for the ADA to hire a qualified research agency to evaluate the quality and cost of closed dental panels in relation to the fee-for-service system.[3]

However, it is generally felt that a civil court would not uphold any action by a dental society that penalized a dentist for earning a living in a closed panel. The main stumbling block to PGPs has been professional resistance to marketing. PGPs need to penetrate the market now so completely dominated by insurance companies and Delta Dental plans, but it is considered unethical for a dentist, acting as an individual or a member of a professional corporation, to solicit patients. It may also in some cases be illegal. If the marketing agency were a nonprofit corporation controlled by the dentists with whom service agreements are made, it would violate the IRS conflict of interest regulations. This would result in the organization's losing its nonprofit status and having its earnings taxed at the corporate level.

A group practice that wishes to initiate a prepaid plan must therefore do so only through a separate third party such as Blue Cross or Blue Shield. Unfortunately, these organizations have no incentive to market PGPs and most of their salespeople are not even familiar with capitation.

This had been the dilemma for some time, but now there seems to be a dramatic reversal of the legal status of advertising that may have a profound impact on PGP marketing. Originally, the Supreme Court stated and reaffirmed in *People v. Duben* (10 N.E. 2d 809 Ill. 229) and *Cherry v. Board of Regents of the State of New York* (44 N.E. 2d 405 N.Y. 148) the states' right to limit advertising by physicians and dentists. However, the court has just decided a case on appeal from the Supreme Court of Arizona, *John R. Bates and Van O'Steen Appellants v. State Bar of Arizona* (76-316 4873, 4895), where it upheld the right of attorneys to advertise their fees for certain services. The State's rule prohibiting this was found in violation of the First Amendment. The court considered six arguments for restricting price advertising—the adverse effect on professionalism, the inherently misleading nature of attorney advertising, the adverse effect on the administration of justice, the undesirable economic effects of advertising, the adverse effect of advertising on the quality of service, and the difficulties of enforcement—and was not persuaded that *any* of them was an acceptable reason for the suppression of *all* advertising by attorneys. However, the court did *not* hold that advertising by attorneys may not be regulated in any way.

It will be interesting to see how this decision affects future litigation concerning advertising and the dental profession. The reasons given by the dental boards as justification for suppressing advertising appear to be very similar to the rationale used by the Arizona bar in relation to attorneys. It is almost certain that First Amendment rights will be claimed in future litigation initiated by the dental profession, and that PGP marketing will eventually be permitted.

Conclusion

The full potential of PGPs has not yet been realized because of the technical, legal, and professional barriers summarized here. It is our conclusion, however, that economic and legal forces currently at work will inexorably lead to a transformation of dental care delivery and that both the dental profession and the public will benefit thereby.

NOTES

1. American Dental Association: *Transactions*, 1967, p. 195.
2. American Dental Association: *Transactions*, 1971, pp. 487–488.
3. Ibid. p. 487.

Workplace Health Hazards: The Responsibilities to Assess, to Report, to Control

Bruce W. Karrh

17

Since the disclosure in 1973 that prolonged exposure to vinyl chloride monomers causes a rare form of liver cancer, occupational health has been transformed into an issue of national concern and debate. The social, moral, and political issues raised are complex and formidable but the need to achieve a higher level of health protection in the workplace is recognized by industry as paramount. As stated by Du Pont Board Chairman Irving S. Shapiro, "There is no more important challenge facing Du Pont, and all of industry, than the broad and expanding issue of occupational health and safety."

The Responsibility to Assess

If an industrial medicine practitioner is to properly assess a site's health conditions, he must first have the resources and the management support to do the job effectively. At Du Pont, as well as at many other companies, the physician's information resources are three: a preemployment medical history and physical examination for each employee, comprehensive medical examinations conducted periodically, and special ongoing medical surveillance programs that monitor persons who could become exposed to highly toxic substances.

A physician needs also to be able to draw on resources that do not necessarily exist at his plant location. Du Pont physicians, for instance, can receive specialized assistance from safety consultants, biostatisticians, industrial hygienists, engineers, and a host of different scientists, doctors. and researchers at the company's centralized Haskell Laboratory for Toxicology and Industrial Medicine. These resources are important to the physician because of the multidimensional nature of long-term, low-level health risks.

Perhaps the most crucial element is management commitment to a safe and healthful work environment. This commitment must permeate the entire line organization from the top management down to first-line supervisors, and must be firm, consistent, and visible. Conversely, it is the physician's duty to counsel management wisely and forthrightly.

If a physician has the resources and the confidence of management, he has the basic components to make positive contributions. In addition, it is essential for him/her to be aware of substances used in the manufacturing process, their toxicity hazards, and how these are controlled. It then depends primarily on his conscientiousness and initiative to implement and sustain a battery of effective programs.

With the new awareness of workplace health hazards, physicians can no longer afford to confine themselves to conducting examinations or to performing emergency services. It was a conscientious plant physician and an industrial hygienist from Haskell Laboratory who first suspected a hazard in a solvent Du Pont uses in the production of a textile fiber. Subsequent laboratory tests showed it to be carcinogenic to rats, a finding that caused the company to initiate extra precautions to protect employees.

Physician work loads now call for more efficient use of technological advances. For instance, at Du Pont physical examination results and epidemiological data are being computerized. At one of the company's largest plants, the health surveillance system has been automated so that an IBM card can show whether an employee's body system is likely to be affected by a particular chemical when he is transferred from one job to another.

The Responsibility to Inform

In its communications with employees on health hazards, a company should operate on the basis of broadly applied principles:

Knowledge: Judgments should be based on the best available knowledge of health hazards and their consequences acquired both internally and from outside the company.

Responsibility: It should be the duty of a company and its chief operating units to acquire adequate operating knowledge through testing and to disseminate this knowledge to all groups with a need to know.

Compliance: Company policy should be to meet or exceed the requirements and implement regulations where specific statutes exist, such as the Toxic Substances Control Act, the Consumer Products Safety Act, and the Occupational Safety and Health Act.

Communications: Employees need to be told of health risks in the workplace and how to deal with these hazards safely in their everyday work practices. Appropriate outside groups—from customers to government agencies—should be notified of potential hazards and actions taken to minimize their impact.

A continual exchange of communication is needed to form a base of credibility and management concern. Otherwise, management ends up speaking in "blasts" when a health hazard bulletin needs to be issued.

Departments and plants should have latitude in choosing how to announce health hazard information to their workers. Du Pont finds the most useful general concept is to give employees basic facts that are technically accurate, complete, and understandable and to provide information about further safe-guards that will be implemented.

Du Pont's system of disclosure—group meetings conducted by supervisors—is far from perfect; it is constantly being evaluated, refined, and updated. But in order to maintain credibility and good relations with employees, customers, and the public, a company's management should be aware that it is not only a matter of ethics to report pertinent health information about products, but that it is good, sound business practice, too. To do less would be both morally irresponsible and, in many instances, economically damaging.

When Should Information Not Be Made Public?

A company must have clear-cut, well-reasoned rules and guidelines for releasing information about health risks. In the case of employees, if the information might affect their well-being or safety, it most certainly should be communicated.

When it comes to communication outside the company, the criteria should be:

—Will this information be useful to these groups (other producers, government agencies, etc.)?

—Will it cause these organizations to take remedial action to protect people who might not otherwise be reached?

—Can these groups disseminate the information on a wider scale to provide additional health and safety benefits?

—Is the communication legally required?

Adhering to such guidelines is, of course, the most ethical and responsible path to follow. But this is far from simple when certain agents may have a clinical latency of from twenty to forty years and when some diseases may result from multifactor interactions. Questions and doubts abound. For instance, how much firm, unimpeachable laboratory evidence should a company have before it reveals a possible health hazard to its employees and the public? Who should get this information? In what form should it be presented? How should the information be reported so the message is understandable yet not unnecessarily alarming? How much effort should be expended to locate former employees who have left the company but who may have worked with hazardous substances at one time? And, when you find them, how do you handle informing members of this group? These are some of the issues that should be addressed before a public announcement is made. They have to be considered diligently and honestly, risks versus benefits have to be evaluated, and, in the end, the overall health interests of employees and the public must dictate the decision. It serves no useful purpose to divulge unsubstantiated risks, especially where the data are questionable. It unnecessarily alarms employees, it breeds public distrust and confusion, and it biases further studies and disclosures.

Somewhere, of course, there is a middle ground. Estimates of risks need not always be supported by batteries of tests and epidemiological data to be valid. For instance, Du Pont has chosen to report health risks based on laboratory tests with animals, epidemiological studies, and even on preliminary lab findings. At times, all these data are felt to be needed to provide conclusive results—but not always. However, I believe that a company should be more inclined to release facts about health risks—*when firm evidence supports the conclusion*—than to withhold them for fear of adverse public reaction or harmful business repercussions.

Who Should Make Decisions?

In the occupational health sphere, with all its complexities, companies must face the fact that decision-making has become a pluralistic process. Workplace health conditions affect employees most certainly, but they also impact surrounding communities, relatives of employees, consumers, and local and federal government entities which may have to contend with and control health risks in the general environment.

All decisions that affect the workplace itself and its profitability must, in the end, be made by the employer. But the employer should seek input from others in making crucial and sensitive decisions about the health of employees. These others include employees, government agencies, consumers, community organizations, and all other appropriate groups.

How best can all these various voices be heard? The solution—and it has been applied with varying degrees of success and confusion already—lies in the political process. In this process all types of opinions coalesce and then are sifted for relevance and practicality. It is an unstable but unavoidable process that more often than not results in surprisingly coherent and durable public decisions.

To make the political process work, all sides need to contribute in a useful manner. Industry must develop sound data which not only cover the cost side of the equation but also the benefit side. The technical, scientific, and medical communities must provide factual data on risks, costs, and benefits. The third major group—the public-at-large, which includes the legislators, regulators, and news media—needs to do its part by avoiding taking positions on emotion, but rather striving to obtain and understand the facts of an issue.

A healthier workplace will require a greater commitment of capital resources. If this results in reduced profits, then so be it. Financial advantage must never be placed above or even equal with human life.

Yet, an employer does not have to concede profitability to achieve a safe and healthy workplace. For one thing, if improved occupational health is a major societal objective—as it most assuredly is—then it should become a cost of doing business and be reflected in the higher cost of products. Second, companies that have followed high health and safety standards over the years have found the result to be more efficient operations. And, finally, profitability need not suffer if an employer exercises shrewd business judgment. Some businesses may have to be discontinued if they cannot be operated within safe health parameters. But the employer who can operate successfully within accepted health guidelines will find that such an achievement may bring more than merely the psychic benefits of acting in a morally responsible manner.

OSHA and Worker Health

The intended goals of the Occupational Safety and Health Act are reasonable and socially desirable. This federal action could galvanize public opinion; it can set a tone of cooperation between all interested parties; it can amass a broad, objective array of scientific knowledge; and it can set priorities for occupational health and safety needs in the United States and direct the best available resources to meet these needs.

From industry's—and from the American public's—standpoint, I believe OSHA has so far fallen far short of its potential to be a positive force in the workplace. It was shackled from the start by a rigid legislative mandate, an ambivalence on whether to concentrate on safety or health or both, and a failure to identify exactly what it should set out to accomplish. The agency's congressional supporters and early administrators also seemed to ignore the practical precept that health protection measures cannot be totally legislated, but must be buttressed by management commitment, the individual worker's acceptance of his own responsibility, and the knowledge that a safe, healthful work environment is a more productive one.

In addition, many of OSHA's past and current practices impede its ability to be truly effective. The intent of OSHA to rely on specification standards rather than on performance criteria has stymied employers by limiting their flexibility and by making certain solutions prohibitively expensive. Too much emphasis has also been placed on enforcement and punitive actions: what has been missing in OSHA so far is a spirit of cooperation. In instances involving small and medium-sized businesses in particular, consultation and resource help—not merely citations for violations—is the prime need.

Perhaps most alarming, from industry's point of view, has been OSHA's tendency toward simplistic solutions to complex health problems. A prime case-in-point is the sweeping new policy proposed for regulating cancer-causing substances in the workplace. The proposed procedures ignore the facts that all carcinogens are not alike and that risks to humans vary considerably according to dosage. This system would be easy for government to administer but wasteful for everyone else.

Nevertheless, OSHA has taken some steps recently that offer glimmers of encouragement. OSHA Director Eula Bingham has gone on record as favoring performance criteria and placing less reliance on specifications. OSHA has also moved to increase consultation services to employers to help locate and solve health and safety problems. This effort is being bolstered by an increase in federal funding to states (up from 50 percent to 90 percent in the federal cost-sharing ratio) for providing consulting services without penalties. Other positive signs include a drive to eliminate nit-picking and concern over marginal problems; an effort to staff the agency and regional offices with more experienced, qualified personnel, including industrial hygienists; and a pledge by Secretary of Labor Ray Marshall to focus on priority problems—"to stop fishing for minnows and start going after whales," as he puts it.

Yet OSHA's likely effect on worker health still looks hazy at best at this time. It is quite possible that the newly enacted Toxic Substances Control Act (P.L. 94-469) will have a more beneficial impact on health in the workplace. It addresses the most current and pressing need in occupational health: the need for more testing so that the public and industry have genuine, objective evidence on which to base future health and safety decisions. The need to know is the chief imperative today.

NOTES

1. F. L. Creech, Jr., and M. W. Johnson, "Angiosarcoma of Liver in the Manufacture of Polyvinyl Chloride," *Journal of Occupational Medicine* 16: 150–151 (1974).

2. *Delays in Setting Workplace Standards for Cancer-Causing and Other Dangerous Substances*, Report to the Congress by the Comptroller General of the United States, HRO 77–71, May 10, 1977.

3. "Eula Bingham: Will She Take the Nonsense Out of OSHA?" *Nations Business* (August 1977): 28–32.

4. *Failure to Meet Commitments Made in the Occupational Safety and Health Act*, Tenth report by the Committee on Government Operations, House report no. 95-710 (Washington, D.C.: USGPO, October 17, 1977).

5. B. W. Karrh "A Company's Duty to Report Health Hazards," presented at the Confer-

ence on Ethical Issues in Occupational Medicine, New York Academy of Medicine, New York, June 22, 1977.

6. Occupational Safety and Health Act of 1970, Public Law 91-596, 91st Congress, S. 2193, December 29, 1970.

7. "An R_X for Ailing OSHA," *Washington Post*, September 12, 1977.

8. Toxic Substances Control Act, Public Law 94-469, 94th Congress, S.3149, October 11, 1976.

The Challenge of Informing Workers of Job-Related Health Hazards

John Friedland

18

With the passing of the Occupational Safety and Health Act (OSHAct) of 1970 (P.L. 91–596), the federal government adopted as policy that, as far as possible, every worker in the United States be assured of safe and healthful working conditions. The first step in eliminating any hazard is, obviously, recognizing it as a hazard. As simplistic as this sounds, however, recognizing health (not safety) hazards is often quite difficult, expensive, and time-consuming.

Symptoms triggered by a brief exposure may take years to develop. During this time the worker may have changed jobs several times and his work records been destroyed, contributing to the difficulty of identifying the hazard. Additionally, the symptoms of occupational illnesses are frequently difficult to differentiate from those of nonoccupational origin, and there may be interaction effects between the two. Also, it is difficult and costly to analyze the consequences of long-term, low-level exposures; for most chemicals we only have evidence about their acute toxic effects. Finally, many workers are exposed to "trade secrets" of unknown composition, and hundreds of new chemicals, many potentially hazardous, are introduced annually.

As a result of these and other factors, estimates of the incidence of occupational illnesses and deaths are inexact. One frequently cited estimate, originally made by the Department of Health, Education, and Welfare in 1972, is of 390,000 occupational disease cases annually and as many as 100,000 deaths.[1] More recently, the Bureau of Labor Statistics (BLS) reported 163,000 job-related illnesses during 1975.[2] However, a study conducted by the University of Washington indicates that the BLS figure may be seriously underestimated.[3]

Excluding skin cancer, the incidence of cancer in the United States is over 600,000 new cases annually. Some knowledgable sources estimate that occupational exposures probably account for over 10 percent of these, while others estimate only 5 percent.[4] This difference of opinion illustrates the difficulty of determining whether diseases are caused by occupational factors, but it is evident that the risk faced by many working Americans is substantial. As a result, employers have both ethical and practical reasons for informing workers about the specific occupational health hazards they face and for allowing them to participate in decision making concerning the handling of those risks.

The Employee's Right to Know

The OSHAct provides, among other things, that employees be apprised of hazards related to promulgated standards, that they be able to observe any required monitoring and/or measuring, have access to the required records, and be promptly notified by the employer if they are being exposed to toxic materials at levels in excess of applicable standards. However, the administration of the law has fallen far short of these objectives. The Labor Department has been hampered by a shortage of properly trained health compliance officers,[5] and has recently recognized that insufficient effort has been directed at controlling serious health hazards.[6]

Questions concerning the legal rights of workers to be informed of known and suspected occupational health hazards, in many instances, are far from settled. The National Research Council's Committee on Public Information in the Prevention of Cancer found "relatively few" statutory responsibilities "assigned to various government agencies . . . concerning the provision of information to the worker."[7] In regard to the legal responsibilities of the employer to inform his employees of occupational health hazards, the director of Yale Law School's Program in Law, Science, and Medicine has stated that the "legally enforceable duty . . . is really a very complicated legal question . . . If an employer actively misrepresents the nature of a risk, workers clearly have a suit, . . . [but] whether [the employer has] to say anything to begin with is . . . more difficult [to determine]."[8]

Despite this uncertainty, the "right to know" is a central theme to many current forces of social change.[9] Its strength is reflected in the vigorous growth of the consumer movement. At the national level, at least nine major laws and amendments requiring disclosure of information to consumers have been enacted. The health professions have become persuaded to pay stricter attention to gaining the informed consent of patients and to include more complete warning information with prescription drugs. Finally, the public's growing disenchantment with management through bureaucracy and distrust of both governmental and private institutions have contributed to the increasingly widespread conviction that individuals' rights are best protected by measures that enable them to protect themselves.

Complementing these social forces is an ethical argument that workers have a right to be informed of occupational health hazards in order to protect their health. Because of the difficulty of determining occupational health hazard risks with certainty, information on suspected or probable risks also needs to be conveyed. The right to know implies an obligation by those having the needed information to communicate it. The duty to disclose, in turn, "entails a moral obligation to continue investigating hazards, and even to shut down production when containment procedures cannot meet some rational minimum standard."[10]

It has been reported that, sometimes, those parties possessing the information needed by workers justify withholding it on grounds that to give the information would create unnecessary anxiety and stress.[11] It is true that, in some instances, increasing the flow of information will raise concerns that are later discovered to be unfounded. However, this problem can be somewhat lessened by having a notification system that has the trust of the workers and that provides the full breadth of pertinent information. To earn their trust, the system will have to overcome worker suspicions that company production and profit automatically take precedence over their health. The system will need to provide, frankly and in a timely fashion, information that not only describes the hazard, but offers a reasonable interpretation of the degree and nature of the risk faced. Equally important is advice about steps that the workers, and their employers, can take to control the risk and to monitor both the work environment and the health status of the employees.

The problem of anxiety, furthermore, does not negate the greater value of the increased choices and enhanced self-determination that full knowledge affords. These choices include the option of refusing, resigning from, or transferring from a hazardous job (the right to voluntarily transfer to a safer job is a short-term negotiating objective of at least one union).[12] Workers who are aware of hazards can also actively monitor their workplace for potentially dangerous conditions and be the source of suggestions and recommendations for reducing exposures, or risks of exposures, to hazardous materials. One such instance, concerning vinyl chloride, has been described by the associate medical director of Exxon Corporation.[13] When workers are aware of their legal and moral rights as well as the technical details of the specific hazards they face (including monitoring and abatement approaches), they can also influence management to voluntarily institute preventive or corrective measures, or negotiate for stronger health provisions in their contracts. If necessary, they can also more effectively seek legally guaranteed protections such as health hazard evaluations by NIOSH or OSHA site visits. Additionally, a work force that is aware of what is not known about the hazards of substances to which they are exposed is more likely politically to encourage a vigorous research effort to close these gaps. As information is obtained through such efforts, workers will be able to substitute informed for uninformed choices.

Finally, an informed work force will be better able to obtain just compensation—through litigation or workers' compensation—for ill effects suffered as a result of occupational health hazards. In fact, lawsuits have already become a serious enough problem that one industry is seeking legislative protection against them.[14]

The Right to Know in Practice

While there appears to be widespread agreement that workers should be informed of occupational health hazards, questions remain as to how this right should be implemented. Particularly important are questions of who should make the determination to inform workers and what parties should be involved in the ensuing communication.

Because the task of determining which substances are hazardous is difficult and because informing workers will require substantial resources, the Committee on Public Information in the Prevention of Cancer recommends "that a single national source, such as DHEW, be charged with making the decision that workers are at risk. This source should be . . . credible to both management and labor."[15] However, because the potential for political intervention in such a process is substantial,[16] representatives (scientific or otherwise) of both labor and management should be included, at least in an advisory capacity, in any working committee charged with this responsibility. This would minimize the possibility that workers would fail to receive appropriate warnings, although perhaps at the expense of a greater number of unnecessary notices received through either official or unofficial channels. But this is an area much subject to honest differences of opinion, and it is better to err on the side of excessive public information.

Once the decision to inform workers has been made, either voluntarily or in response to a directive, there are a wide variety of resources including those of management, industrial medical departments, government, labor unions, peer leaders among the workers, public interest groups, professional associations, educational institutions, and the press that can be involved. Many factors affect the decision on which of these resources should be used.

First, the message received will vary with the perceived integrity of its source and with how successfully the message attracts the target group's attention. Second, the number of people reached by a message will increase with multiple exposures of the message and with the use of multiple informational sources. These measures increase the probability that the message will be available when individual target group members are receptive.[17] Third, the dissemination of health information can proceed "from the top down" (where facts are disseminated by experts having high credibility to relatively passive recipients) or "from the bottom up" (where the objective is to get the workers quickly involved in exercises to improve their work environment and to build on these accomplishments and behavioral changes to create an increased desire and interest for information).[18] Finally, although the determination of what constitutes an occupational health hazard can (perhaps) be considered to be within the province of scientific inquiry, an equally important part of the message to be transmitted to workers involves recommended actions to be taken in response to the hazard.

The formulation of action recommendations and the implementation of these or other actions are social and political issues that appropriately should involve broad participation.[19] An inference that can be drawn from these four points is that each of the available resource groups, with their differing orientations, can contribute to the overall task of disseminating occupational health information to the work force. This conclusion coincides with the recommendation of the Committee on Public Information in the Prevention of Occupational Cancer that "sources in addition to OSHA, NIOSH, and employers should be used [in communicating health hazards information to workers]. Supplemental sources that offer promise include labor unions, extension services of the land grant colleges and other adult education activities, state, county, and municipal health departments and community oriented public service health groups."[20]

Not everyone concurs with this recommendation. One dissenting opinion is that "the one thing, and the only thing [needed to inform workers] is management's commitment . . . Yes, you already have management's commitment to all of this."[21] In respect to this dissenting position, it is fair to note that some companies have by themselves budgeted large amounts of money into occupational health hazard research and have voluntarily reduced acceptable exposure levels to toxic substances.[22] But others have not.[23] Furthermore, there have been more than a few accounts suggesting that industry's self-regulation and compliance have in general fallen far short of this.[24] Among the charges levied in these accounts are management constraints on the communication of toxicologic information, biased manipulation of data, misleading statements, application of biological controls for hazards which are themselves hazardous to workers, callousness, and carelessness.

Although some will dismiss these charges as unfounded and/or politically motivated, the very magnitude of the list of grievances must cast a note of caution on any such dismissal. In addition, although a number of companies have publicly defended their efforts to protect and inform their employees, or have had their efforts favorably reviewed by others,[25] "insiders" such as the head of industrial medicine for Kaiser Industries Corporation have noted that public responses from industry to these public charges have been practically nonexistent.[26] More recently, the editor of Occupational Health and Safety Letter asserted that industry's typical reaction when approached for its side of a story about an occupational health problem is either "defensive, stonewall, [or] no comment."[27] The public record, to date, simply does not support endorsing management as the sole source of occupational health information for workers. Where the schism between labor and management is not so wide as to prevent cooperation, however, management and company medical personnel can be an important participant in this offer.

It should also be noted that the other resources are still quite limited. Only a few unions have full-time staff devoted to health matters, public interest groups face budgeting constraints, and the occupational health education and training efforts of government agencies have been limited in funding and staffing. These limitations do serve to increase the potential positive role that management can assume.

Where the necessary credibility with the work force does not exist, management and company medical officers should immediately initiate the unavoidably long process of demonstrating their commitment to the health of the workers through their daily actions, strictly complying with regulations having to do with reporting occupational disease and establishing a direct, unfiltered channel of communication between the medical officer and top levels of management.[28] It has also been suggested that the field of occupational medicine take positive steps to improve its credibility, including initiation of a "confidential review process . . . to consider complaints of management obstruction . . . (and) a public censure process for corporations determined by due process to have violated ethical medical practice."[29]

In conclusion, occupational health hazards are a major problem for workers in America. For social, ethical, and (increasingly) legal reasons, workers have a right and a need to be apprised of those hazards and to play an active role in defining what is to be society's response to them. A substantial number of activities (some listed below) have been undertaken in the past few years to assist meeting these needs. But more remains to be done. Even the General Accounting Office, one of the government's commonly recognized "watchdog" agencies, has recommended that the Department of Labor allocate more funding to occupational health information, education, and training activities.[30]

A number of suggestions have been offered concerning activities that could be undertaken to work toward meeting the informational needs of workers about occupational health hazards. These suggestions include the development of a national clearinghouse on hazard facts, methodologies for informing workers, and available resources; the development of incentives aimed at encouraging voluntary employee group compliance with safe work practices; training and utilizing staff of local public health agencies and university extension programs to meet the educational needs of workers in small businesses; and offering government funding to public interest groups. Whichever approach or approaches are eventually adopted, the ongoing discovery of occupational hazards, in the form of both newly introduced and long-used agents, and the need to reinforce and update previously transmitted data assure that a continued escalation of effort in this area will be necessary.

Partial Listing of Sources of Information about Programs to Inform and Educate Workers about Occupational Health Hazards

1.   Nicholas Ashford, Crisis in the Workplace (Cambridge, Mass: M.I.T. Press, 1975), especially pp. 482–487 and 490–495.

2.   Office of Training and Education, Occupational Safety and Health Administration, U.S. Department of Labor, Washington, D. C. Descriptions of current training contracts and programs supported by OSHA.

3.   Technical Publications Development Section, Technical Information

Development Branch, National Institute for Occupational Safety and Health, U.S. Department of Health, Education, and Welfare, Cincinnati, Ohio. Publishes guides for targeted small businesses on health and safety guidelines and applicable OSHA regulations, and a series of work practice manuals for workers in specific occupations. NIOSH also issues alerts (through "current intelligence bulletins") to business, labor, government, public interest, and scientific representatives when information on potentially dangerous chemicals is received.

4. Bert Cottine, et al., *Winning at the Occupational Safety and Health Review Commission: A Worker's Handbook on Enforcing Safety and Health Standards* (Washington, D. C.: Health Research Group, 1975).

5. Andrea Hricko and Melanie Brunt, *Working for Your Life: A Woman's Guide to Job Health Hazards* (Berkeley, Calif.; Labor Occupational Health Program and Health Research Group, 1976). Includes lists of groups, publications, and films available to assist workers.

6. *How to Use OSHA: A Worker's Guide to the Occupational Safety and Health Administration* (Cambridge, Mass.: Occupational Safety and Health Project, Urban Planning Aid, 1975).

7. Safety and Health Project, University of Wisconsin- Extension, School for Workers, Madison, Wisc., Pamphlets, films, courses, and training aids.

8. Labor Occupational Health Program, Center for Labor Research and Education, University of California, Berkeley. Newsletter, publications, courses, films, and a variety of services such as assistance in designing and implementing health and safety programs. The January, 1977 issue of the Program's newsletter (*LOHP Monitor*) reviews many of their activities.

9. "Organized Labor Campaign for Improved Health Found Hampered by Shortages of Resources," *Daily Labor Report* (Sept. 9, 1976): A4–5.

10. Virginia Reinhart, "A Model Union Program," *Job Safety and Health* (August 1977): 14–19.

11. "Paperworkers Health Evaluated," *Job Safety and Health* (August 1977): 42–43.

12. "Leukemia Deaths of Some Rubber Workers Prompt Study of Possible Connection to Job," *Wall Street Journal* (July 22, 1976): 34.

13. "OCAW Urges Local Unions to Report Safety Cases to Union Central Office," *Daily Labor Report* (Sept. 5, 1974): A11–A12.

14. "Safety and Health Provisions the OSHAct of 1970," *Monthly Labor Review* (Sept. 1975): 40–43.

15. *Major Collective Bargaining Agreements: Safety and Health Provisions*, U.S. Dept. of Labor, Bureau of Labor Statistics, bulletin 1425-16, 1976.

16.   David Wegman, M.D. et al., "Health Hazard Surveillance by Industrial Workers," *American Journal of Public Health* (January 1975): 26–30.

17.   *Occupational Safety and Health Training Grants, 1976–1977.* United States Department of Health, Education, and Welfare, NIOSH, Division of Training and Manpower Development, Cincinnati, Ohio. November, 1976.

18.   "Labor Agency to Rush Rules for Business on Disclosing Chemical Peril to Workers," *Wall Street Journal* (April 29, 1977): 14.

19.   U.S. Department of Labor, OSHA, (29 CFR Part 1970), *Identification, Classification and Regulation of Toxic Substances Posing a Potential Occupational Carcinogenic Risk.* Note of Proposed Rulemaking, pp. 126, 167–173, U.S. Government Printing Office: 1977, 0-247-285/6600.

20.   U.S. Department of Labor, Office of Information, "OSHA Proposes New Comprehensive Regulation on Workplace Cancer Hazards" October 3, 1977.

21.   "Bill Offered in Senate to Allow IRS Records to be Used for Cancer Warnings" *Daily Labor Report* (April 6, 1977): A4–A5.

22.   "The Problems with OSHA's Cancer Proposal," *Business Week* (October 24, 1977): 38.

23.   "Cotton Dust: Textile Workers and PIRG File Suit to Compel Labor Department to Modify Existing Standards," *Daily Labor Report* (January 12, 1976).

24.   "OSHA Petitioned to Ban Chloroform Exposure," *Job Safety and Health* (July 1977): 2.

25.   "Sterility, Cancer Risk," *AFL-CIO News* (August 27, 1977): 3.

26.   Thomas Mancuso, M.D., *Help for the Working Wounded* (Washington D.C., Industrial Association of Machinists and Aerospace Workers, 1976).

NOTES

1. Nicholas A Ashford, *Crisis in the Workplace* (Cambridge, Mass.: MIT Press, 1975), pp. 4, 93; and Paul Brodeur, *Expendable Americans* (New York: Viking Press, 1974), p. 158.

2. "BLS Reports Drop in Job-Related Injuries, Illnesses, and Deaths," *Daily Labor Report,* December 8, 1976, pp. B3–B4.

3. Cited in Ashford, *Crisis in the Workplace,* pp. 96–97.

4. *Public Information in the Prevention of Occupational Cancer,* Proceedings of a Symposium, December 2–3, 1976, Committee on Public Information in the Prevention of Occupational Cancer, National Research Council, National Academy of Sciences, Washington, April 1977 (hereafter, PIPOC-Symposium), Umberto Saffiotti, p. 36; and J. Higginson, "A Hazardous Society? Individual versus Community Responsibilities in Cancer Prevention," *Amercian Journal of Public Health,* 66: 359–366 (1976).

5. Morton Corn and Earl Health, "OSHA Response to Occupational Health Personnel Needs and Resources," *American Industrial Hygiene Association Journal,* 38: 11–17 (January 1977).

6. Walter Mossberg, "Safety Agency Will Tighten Regulations on Health Hazards, Drop Trivial Rules," *Wall Street Journal,* May 19, 1977, p. 48.

7. *Informing Workers and Employers About Occupational Cancer,* Committee on Public Information in the Prevention of Occupational Cancer, National Research Council, National Academy of Sciences, Washington 1977 (hereafter, PIPOC-Report), p. 13. Nevertheless the committee concludes that the laws do provide a clear "legal basis for providing public information for the prevention of occupational cancer," p. 15.

8. PIPOC-Symposium, Angela Holder, pp. 57–61. Also see the chapter by Blum in this volume.

9. Harold Magnuson, M.D., "The Right to Know," *Archives of Environmental Health,* (January-February 1977): 40–44.

10. *PIPOC-Symposium,* Dr. Joseph Fletcher, p. 55, also see Leroy Walters, p. 190.

11. *PIPOC-Symposium,* Andrea Hricko, Labor Occupational Health Program, p. 69, and David Wegman, Assistant Professor of Occupational Medicine, Harvard University, School of Public Health, p. 74. For a specific example, see "Nader Group Says Rohm and Haas Company Supressed Data," *Wall Street Journal,* October 3, 1974, p. 12.

12. *PIPOC-Symposium,* Andrea Hricko, p. 87.

13. Ibid., Dr. Robert Eckardt, p. 49.

14. Jack Anderson and Les Whitten, "Asbestos Firms Seek Way Out of Lawsuits," *Boston Globe,* October 5, 1977.

15. PIPOC-Report, p. 11.

16. The "OSHA-1972 Nixon Campaign" Memorandum is a near-perfect example of this possibility. See Ashford, *Crisis in the Workplace,* pp. 538, 543–544.

17. *PIPOC-Symposium,* Brenda Dervin, Assistant Professor of Communications, University of Washington, pp. 109, 113.

18. Ibid., Herbert Simons, Professor of Speech, Temple University, pp. 115–119.

19. Ibid., Dr. Umberto Saffiotti, pp. 37–38, Joseph Wagoner, Division of Field Studies and Clinical Investigations, NIOSH, p. 8, and Leroy Walters, p. 189.

20. PIPOC-Report, p. 25.

21. *PIPOC-Symposium,* Dr. Robert Magor, Manager of Industrial Hygiene, Polaroid Corporation, p. 99.

22. See for instance, "Protecting the Health of DuPont Employees Is a Costly Proposition," *Wall Street Journal,* June 28, 1976, pp. 1, 19; and Barry Kramer, "Vinyl-Chloride Risks Were Known by Many before First Deaths," *Wall Street Journal,* October 2, 1974, pp. 1, 22.

23. At least one eminent defender of the free enterprise system has argued that the *voluntary* diversion of corporate resources by management to accomplish social objectives, within which I would include the protection of worker health as long as management can successfully externalize most related costs, is inappropriate. See Milton Friedman, "The Social Responsibility of Business is to Increase Profits," *New York Times Magazine,* September 13, 1970.

24. See Brodeur, *Expendable Americans,* William Randall and Stephen Solomon, *Building 6: The Tragedy at Bridesberg* (Boston: Little Brown, 1977); U.S. Congress Hearings of Subcommittee on Oversight and Investigations, House Committee on Interstate and Foreign Commerce, May 28 and September 20, 1976, Serial No. 94-141, *Environmental Causes of Cancer,* pp. 8–29, 190, 296–199, and 304–313; William Morton, M.D., "The Responsibility to Report Occupational Health Risks," *Journal of Occupational Medicine:* 19: 258–260 (April 1977); "A Sterility Scare Sends OSHA Scurrying," *Business Week,* September 12, 1977, pp. 45–48; "Industrial Sterility," *Newsweek,* August 29, 1977, p. 69;

Jon Swan, "No News From the Press Room" *Columbia Journalism Review* (May-June 1977): 31–36; Gail Bronson, "Confrontation of DuPont, Health Agency Is Sparked by Employee's Cancer Worries," *Wall Street Journal*, February 11, 1977, p. 4; Barry Kramer, "Vinyl-Chloride Risks Were Known by Many Before First Deaths," *Wall Street Journal*, October 2, 1974, pp. 1, 22; "New Lead-Disease Data Spur U.S. To Ask Smelters to Tighten Controls on Exposure," *Wall Street Journal*, February 23, 1976, p. 16; "Exposure to Toxic Substances by Millions of Unaware Workers Warned at Hearing," *Wall Street Journal*, April 28, 1977, p. 8; "Nader Group Says Rohm and Haas Company Suppressed Data," *Wall Street Journal*, October 3, 1974, p. 12; and "Rohm and Haas Finds Excess Cancer Rate at Bristol, Pennsylvania Plant," *Wall Street Journal*, July 22, 1976, p. 34.

25. See, "DuPont Mobilizes against The Risk of Occupational Cancer," *DuPont Management Bulletin*, April 1976 (reproduced in *Environmental Causes of Cancer*, pp. 99–104); *PIPOC-Symposium*, David Wegman, pp. 74–75; "From the B.F. Goodrich Company— Vinyl Chloride and Cancer: A Study in Prevention." Job Safety and Health, February 1977, pp. 20–28; W. H. Weiss, "The Safety-Minded Company," *Job Safety and Health*, September 1976, pp. 28–33; and "Protecting the Health of DuPont Employees is a Costly Proposition," *Wall Street Journal*, June 28, 1976, pp. 1, 19.

26. Clifford H. Keene, M.D., "The Credibility of Occupational Medicine," *Journal of Occupational Medicine:* 16: 309–312 (May 1974).

27. *PIPOC-Symposium*, Gerhson Fishbein, p. 93.

28. Keene, "The Credibility of Occupational Medicine," pp. 311–312.

29. William Morton, "Responsibility to Report Occupational Health Risks," *Journal of Occupational Medicine*, 19(4): 260 (April 1977).

30. "GAO Advocates Faster Development of Health Standards in Workplace." *Daily Labor Report* (May 16, 1977): A5–A8.

Revealing the Invisible Tort: The Employer's Duty to Warn

John D. Blum

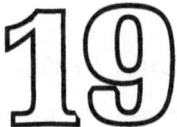

Despite warning signs about asbestos dust and despite nearly five decades of evidence, some supervisors in that Johns-Manville [Lampoc, California] plant were telling workers as recently as two years ago that the stories about asbestos causing disease were just rumors.

> Columbia Journalism Review
> September–October 1977, p. 43.

A little-known pesticide called dibromochloroprane is causing shock waves through the chemical industry and the health community ... Embarrassed industry and government officials have been forced to admit that a study sponsored by Dow and Shell pinpointed the compound's dangers as long ago as 1961.

> Business Week
> September 12, 1977, p. 47.

Unfortunately, these incidents are not unique: far too often information about hazardous health conditions in the workplace reaches workers only after serious injuries have occurred.[1] While widespread consensus exists about the desirability of disseminating reliable and timely health hazard information, there is presently no agreement about what sorts of information should be provided to workers: it is unclear just what responsibilities employers have in informing employees about health hazards confronted on the job.

The issue of informing workers involves a number of complex problems. Frequently it is hard to determine at what level exposure to a toxic agent becomes dangerous to human beings. As a result, effective regulations are difficult to develop. In some instances industry and labor may reject standards, even if scientifically sound because of the high cost of compliance and the danger of fostering unnecessary concern among workers. Still, there are enough widely recognized health hazards that employees should be notified of routinely, and whether this will in fact occur depends upon the responsibilities placed by law upon employers.

Currently there is no independently recognized duty on the part of an employer to notify workers about exposure to harmful conditions at the workplace. The area is, however, in a process of development in both the common and statutory law.

General Safety Responsibility and the Duty to Warn

Under the common law a well-established duty exists on the part of employers to provide a safe working environment. This duty has been affirmed and partially defined in a number of state court cases: for example in *Shimp v. New Jersey Bell Telephone Co.* (368 A2d 408, N.J. Super Ct. 1976), a New Jersey court stated "an employee has a right to work in a safe environment, the employer is under an affirmative duty to provide a work area that is free from unsafe working conditions." However, the degree of effort an employer must exert for this purpose will vary with the circumstances and industry involved.[2] In no case is he an insurer against accidents of illness, especially where the employee's behavior constitutes contributory negligence or assumption of a known risk. Further, the employer is not liable when a worker is injured because of the details and risks of a particular task.

Arising from the general duty to provide a safe working environment is the responsibility to warn about dangerous conditions in the workplace if the adverse condition present in the work environment is not readily apparent to the worker.

On the other hand, if a danger is clearly recognized by employees as an obvious one, the employer may not be held liable for failure to point it out.[3]

The duty to warn also varies with all the circumstances surrounding a given industry: "whether a warning or instruction is necessary may depend upon the age, intelligence, and experience of the employees as well as on the nature of the danger, the character of the work and the surrounding conditions and circumstances."[4] In the case of *Dowler v. New York, Chicago & St. Louis*

Railroad Co. (125 N.E.2d 41 (Ill. 1955)) the court ruled that the danger of burn injury from creosote is not a matter of common knowledge (as is the danger from gasoline) and thus found liability for failure to warn. If the injured employee had has a great deal of experience working with creosoted materials, then the ruling may well have been otherwise. It should be noted that while the duty to warn is variable, it is not affected by local custom: the fact that other industries in a given area do not provide warnings is not a valid defense.

In order for the employer to be held legally responsible for warning employees about hazardous conditions, it must be demonstrated that the employer was the source of the injury.[5] Problems do arise in determining what health hazards an employer should be aware of. Under the doctrine of constructive knowledge (knowledge that an individual has the opportunity to possess by exercise of ordinary care), an employer is held responsible for knowing about hazardous conditions that could be ascertained by reasonable inspection, testing, or monitoring efforts.[6] Under the common law doctrine of assumption of skill, knowledge of dangerous conditions at the workplace is automatically attributed to the employer, generally if they could not be readily ascertained by the employee.[7] The rationale underlying this is that employees act on the employer's orders and so the employer has a special responsibility to ensure that the duties he assigns do not place workers in perilous situations they are unaware of.

Results of Medical Exams

Also emanating from the general duty of the employer for the safety of the worker is a duty to inform about the adverse results of medical examinations given under company auspices. While there is no legal responsibility on the part of an employer to provide medical exams, adverse results must be communicated if such exams are in fact given. This requirement stems from a basic common law doctrine that creates a responsibility of due care on those who induce others to rely on their actions for self-protection.[8] In order for the employer to be held liable under this doctrine, it must be demonstrated that he had actual or constructive knowledge of the results. Generally, any information contained in employee health records or discovered by a physician, employee, or agent is held to be known by the employer.[9] The case of *Coffee v. McDonnell Douglas* (503 P2d 1366 (1972)) illustrates the principle that the employer also has an affirmative duty to consider an employee's physical condition prior to making work assignments. However, the scope of that responsibility cannot extend beyond what are considered to be reasonable medical findings in a given instance. Thus, even if corporate physicians fail to diagnose a certain condition, liability will not arise provided due care was exercised in conducting the examination and the medical conclusions were reasonable.[10] Also it must be shown that the employee was unaware of his condition.[11]

The employer's liability for failure to disclose the existence of an adverse physical condition discovered through a medical examination can extend to injuries involving a third party. In *Wojcik v. Aluminum Co. of America* (183 NYS2d 351 (1959)) the defendant corporation negligently failed to inform one of its workers about the existence of tuberculosis, revealed in an x-ray; thus the worker failed to seek necessary treatment, aggravating the condition. His wife sued as a third party when she contracted the contagious disease from him, and the company was found liable for her injury.

A Note on Workmen's Compensation

Injuries arising out of the three common law duties—the duty to maintain safe working conditions, the duty to warn about dangerous workplace conditions, and the duty to inform workers about adverse results of medical examination—would all be compensable events under state workmen's compensation laws. Workmen's compensation often is the exclusive remedy in actions between employee and employer, precluding outside judicial action. While separate suits may be maintained against other parties, for instance third-party physicians, many states have expressly excluded employer-employee litigation when the action falls under workmen's compensation coverage.[12]

However variances in workmen's compensation laws among the states have always resulted in some jurisdictions' allowing for certain kinds of independent actions. For example, New York State allowed a separate civil suit in *Wojcik* (supra), holding that workmen's compensation was not the sole remedy for such a case. In some states courts have ruled that intentional wrongdoing or serious misconduct on the part of an employer will give rise to a civil suit, either as an alternative to workmen's compensation or cumulative to a right of statutory compensation.[13] It could be argued that an employer's action in covering up information about hazardous conditions in the workplace constitutes an intentional tort, thus leading to separate judicial action outside workmen's compensation in states allowing for alternative legal resolution.

Another way independent suits can be maintained is through the use of the dual capacity doctrine. Under the theory of dual capacity, "an employer normally shielded from tort liability by the exclusive remedy principle may become liable in tort to his own employees if he occupies in addition to his capacity as an employer, a second capacity that confers on him obligations independent of those imposed on him as an employer."[14] Consider a situation where a manufacturer-employer fails to inform his employee about a hazardous piece of equipment and the employee is subsequently injured as a result of his ignorance. In such a case the injury would be compensable under workmen's compensation but a separate lawsuit may be filed on the basis of a failure to warn emanating from a products liability doctrine.

Products Liability Doctrine and the Duty to Warn

A possible grounds for an employer's legal duty to warn can be developed under the products liability doctrine. This principles make a manufacturer liable to a user of his product if the product is defective, if the manufacturer has knowledge (actual, constructive) of the defect, and if the defect causes injury.[15] This is an issue of strict liability; that is, the question of negligence does not arise. Products liability actions tend to be divided into two basic types, those in which the product is flawed because of a miscarriage in the manufacturing process, and those in which the product was produced according to plan but flawed in design. In the latter case, the failure to provide a warning has been treated in and of itself as a defect.[16] In cases where the product in question is unavoidably unsafe because of limitations in scientific knowledge, warnings become essential and failure to provide them stands as grounds for classifying the product as unreasonably dangerous.[17]

While the products liability cases embody a duty to warn of unavoidably unsafe products, these suits are between manufacturer and worker, not employee and employer. The employer who has purchased a machine that causes an injury may be named in a products liability suit but primary responsibility rests with the manufacturer. In cases where liability stems from the failure to warn, however, an employer-purchaser rather than a manufacturer may be found liable. The manufacturer's duty to warn may be fulfilled by providing detailed instruction and warning to the employer. The employer then has a duty to pass on the manufacturer's warning or instructions to employees concerning an unavoidably unsafe product.[18]

Products liability places a more extensive duty on the manufacturer in relation to his employees.[19] Frequently, injury resulting from a failure to warn will be exclusively covered under workmen's compensation, but products liability actions do not lie under this kind of legislation. Thus, under the dual capacity doctrine (supra) a worker who has been injured because of the failure to warn can bring an action against the employer on the grounds of products liability.

The Employer's Duty to Warn under Statute

Specific responsibilities concerning provision of health information to employees are defined in the regulations issued pursuant to the federal Occupational Safety and Health Act (P.L. 91-596). In addition, state labor law codes, workmen's compensation acts, and special occupational health and safety acts also contain such requirements, some comprehensive in scope.

Occupational Safety and Health Act

Under OSHA employers have a general duty to provide employees with a workplace that is free from recognized hazards and to follow whatever safety regulations are issued pursuant to the law. Violations of an OSHA standard will result in the issuance of a citation requiring the abatement of a given condition. Failure to correct may lead to a financial penalty or criminal sanction, depending upon the severity of the violation. Private causes of action are not possible for violation of an OSHA standard.[20]

OSHA requires employers to notify employees if they have been exposed to a harmful or toxic substance at a limit exceeding established exposure levels. The general policy of the Occupational Safety and Health Administration is that workers should be notified regardless of whether their exposure to a harmful or toxic substance exceeded established levels. The required frequency of notification will vary depending upon the speed with which safety measures would have to be instituted to protect workers from a given exposure.

Emergency temporary standards (ETS) for Dibromo-3-chloropropone (DBCP) illustrate the current comprehensive information requirements within a given standard.[21] Employers are required to notify OSHA when they are using this chemical to allow the agency to assemble a profile concerning the safety capabilities of the industry in question and the nature of the affected workforce. Employers are further required to monitor the level of exposure for each employee coming in contact with the chemical. Where worker exposures are above the set acceptable level, monitoring is required on a monthly rather than quarterly basis. Employees are to be notified in writing of the monitoring results and, if the permissible exposure levels are exceeded, the company must describe what corrective actions it will take.

In addition, medical surveillance is required for each employee who is or will be exposed to DBCP. A specified medical examination and tests are to be conducted prior to initial work assignments and whenever the worker is exposed to unsafe levels of this chemical. Records of the monitoring results are to be kept and made available to employees who request to examine and copy them. Also, employers are required to train employees in the specific hazard and the methods best suited for guarding against injuries and to provide appropriate warnings to continually remind workers of potential danger.[22]

Toxic Substances Control Act

The federal Toxic Substances Control Act (TSCA), P.L. 94-469, states:

> Any person who manufactures, processes or distributes in commerce a chemical substance or mixture and who obtains information which reasonably supports the conclusion that such substance or mixture presents a substantial risk of injury to health or the environment shall immediately inform the administrator (of EPA) of such information.

According to recently promulgated guidelines, warning signs that would necessitate a report involve effects on human health, adverse scientific study results, serious environmental danger, and specific incidents of environmental contamination. For example, under the human health category is included, "any instance of cancer, gene mutations, or birth defects. Any instance of toxicity that results in death or serious or prolonged incapacitation (other than due to gross use)."[23] The information concerning potential harm owing to a chemical does not have to be conclusive so long as it is reasonable to demonstrate the risk.

The information requirement of TSCA does not extend to an employer obligation to notify employees. Presumably, the administrator of EPA who receives notice of a verifiable danger will make the information public, and thus workers will be so informed (at least indirectly). Also, information concerning the adverse nature of a chemical will be passed on to OSHA, and the latter agency can develop special information requirements.

State Law

Basically, whatever duty the employer has under state law to inform his employees about hazardous work conditions stems from the general common law responsibility to provide a safe working environment. Still, in a growing number of states legislation has been enacted that lays down (to a widely varying degree) specific employer requirements to inform workers about health risks. Much of the state legislation and regulations are developed pursuant to the creation of state plans under OSHA.

The California Occupational Health and Safety Act of 1973 is one of the more comprehensive state industrial safety laws, by and large paralleling OSHA.[24] It requires employers to post information regarding employee protections and employer obligations under the occupational safety law. Notice of citations issued by the Division of Industrial Safety are to be posted at or near the place of violation. Employees shall have the opportunity to observe the monitoring or measurement processes and are to be allowed access to records of exposure to toxic or harmful substances. The law specifically requires that employees who have been exposed to dangerous substances in excess of exposure standards be so informed, and that they further be notified of what corective actions are being taken.

While the California law is modeled on the federal law it represents a significant transfer of authority in the occupational health regulation area. As more states receive approval for their occupational health plans pursuant to OSHA, enforcement of (in some cases, development of) informational standards in the workplace will become the responsibility of state government.

Conclusions

The law is moving toward an independent duty on the part of the employer to supply workers with information about adverse health conditions, separate from a cause of action for a given physical injury. From the general safety requirement of the common law emanates a legal duty to warn about harmful or dangerous conditions in the workplace and to provide the results of adverse physical exams given under employer auspices. Presently, this does not stand as an independent cause of action: it can be raised only where the omission has lead to a worker injury.

Products liability may serve to create a duty to inform stemming from a manufacturer's responsibility to inform workers about the possible hazards of unavoidably unsafe equipment. The effects of products liability actions may be especially important where the dual capacity doctrine allows for civil suits against employer-manufacturers.

The statutory obligations to notify workers exposed to harmful substances under both OSHA and state law are applicable only under a given standard. Under current statutory law, the employer has no general duty to notify employees when they are exposed to a harmful or toxic substance, and the process of determining standards is both slow and controversial.

On the basis of the legal assessment made here, eight recommendations can be made with the goal of developing a duty to warn about workplace health hazards in both the common and statutory law.

(1) State and federal courts should recognize failure to inform workers about a hazardous condition as giving rise to an independent civil action, not related to another injury.

(2) The failure to warn about a workplace health hazard should be seen as an intentional tort.

(3) Products liability should be generally recognized as compelling warnings about hazards in the manufacturing process.

(4) A general statutory obligation should be required under OSHA so that if "reasonable" evidence exists that a given substance is carcinogenic the employer must automatically inform workers who may be exposed even if no standard has been developed.

(5) Employees should have a general right of access to all personal medical records held by their employers.

(6) The National Institute of Occupational Safety and Health (NIOSH) should be allowed access to employee health records for purposes of conducting epidemiological studies of occupational illness without having to obtain informed consent from each worker. NIOSH study results based on employee records should be strictly protected, released only in aggregate form.

(7) The Toxic Substance Control Act should be amended so that notice of a potentially dangerous chemical be provided to workers at the same time such information is given to the administrator of EPA.

(8) Finally, the extent of required warnings should depend upon the type of industry involved. Employers dealing with toxic substances that are not readily apparent as such should have responsibility to provide detailed and frequent warnings.

NOTES

1. Currently, HEW is being sued by 400 asbestos workers for failure to inform. See *Performance of the OSHA Administration*, U.S. Congress, Subcommittee of the Committee on Government Operations Hearings, 95th Congress, April 27-28, 1977.

2. *Faulks, v. Fischer* 37 A2d 574 (Pa. 1944).

3. Prosser, William L. *The Law of Torts*, Chap. 13, sec. 80, 1971; see also, *Mellor v. Ten Sleep Cattle Company* 550 P2d 500 (1976); *Haley v. Allied Chemical Corporation* 231 N.E. 2d 549 (Mass. 1967); *Cabrera v. Delta Brands, Inc.* 538 S.W.2d 795 (1976); 56 C.J.S. sec. 284, p. 1048.

4. 56 C.J.S. sec. 284, p. 1046.

5. 56 C.J.S. sec. 286, p. 1050; see also *Shuman v. Mashburn* 223 S.E.2d 268 (1976).

6. 56 C.J.S. sec. 286, p. 1050; see also *Maty v. Grasselli Chemical Co.* 98 F2d 877 (3rd Cir, 1938).

7. 7 C.J.S., p. 136; see also *Genesco Inc. v. Greeson* 125 S.E.2d 786 (Ga. App. 1962); *Mid-Continent Pipe Company v. Price* 225 P2d 176 (Ok. 1950); and *Burton v. Wadley Southern Railroad Company* 103 S.E. 881 (Ga. Appl. 1920).

8. American Law Institute, *Restatement of the Law of Torts* 2d vol. 2, sec. 325; and *Union Carbide & Carbon Corp. v. Stapleton* 237 F2d (1956).

9. See *DuPont E.I. DuPont De Nemours & Co. v. Brown* 102 F2d 786 (1939); *Blue Bell Globe Mfg. Co. v. Lewis* 27 SO2d 900 (Miss. 1946); and *Waller v. Southern Pacific Co.* 424 P2d 937 (Ca. 1967). A physician acting on behalf of a corporation in providing physical examinations has been held personally liable for failure to inform an examined employee about an adverse medical condition. See *Vela v. Wise* (Cal. Super. Ct. Contra Costa Co. Docket no. 11603, n.1, 1973). If a physician can be found liable for failure to inform under the master-servant doctrine (one which holds the employer liable for the torts of an employee), and employer could in turn be held vicariously liable for such failure.

10. *Jines v. General Electric Co.* 303 F2d 76 9th Cir. (1962).

11. *DuPont* (supra).

12. See J. D. Blum "Growing Liabilities in Corporate Clinics," in Richard H. Egdahl, ed., *Background Papers on Industry's Changing Role in Health Care Delivery* (New York: Springer-Verlag, 1977); *Bradshaw v. Iowa Methodist Hospital* 241 Iowa 375 (1960); and *Lotspeich v. Chance Vought Aircraft* 369 S.W.2d 705 (Texas 1973).

13. *Douglas v. E. J. Gallo Winery*, 137 Cal. Rptr. 797 (1977); and *Magliulo v. Superior Court*, 121 Cal. Rptr. 621 (1975).

14. Lawson, *Law of Workmen's Compensation*, vol. 2a sec. 7280.

15. Supra at note 8, sec 402(a).

16. John W. Wade "On the Nature of Strict Tort Liability for Products," 44 *Mississippi Law Journal* 825 (November 1973).

17. See *Borel v. Fiberboard Paper Products Corp.* 493 F2d 1076 (1973); and *Phillips v. Kimwood Machine Co.* 525 P2d 1033 (1974).

18. J. T. Elser "Asbestosis: It's Impact upon Products Liability and Workmen's Compensation 1975," *Insurance Law Journal* 459 (August 1975). An analogy can be drawn between the employer's duty to warn and that of a physician who is obligated to pass a manufacturer's drug warnings to a patient. (This is subject to some confusion with the package insert controversy.)

19. Ibid. and *Douglas* (supra).

20. *Russell v. Bartley and Barton and Bell* (494 F2d 334 [6th Cir. 1974]).

21. 42 F.R. 45535 (September 9, 1977).

22. Ibid.

23. 42 F.R. 45365 (September 9, 1977).

24. Cal. Labor Code, sec. 6300, et seq.

Appendix

Conference Participants Quoted

"Employee and Employer Decisions About Health:
Informational Issues"
Boston University Center for Industry and Health Care
Boston: November 4–5, 1977

Gregory J. Ahart, Director, Human Resources Division, General Accounting
Office, Washington, D.C.

Lawrence K. Altman, M.D., Medical Writer, Science News Department, *New
York Times*, New York, New York (on leave)

George J. Annas, J.D., Director, Center for Law and Health Sciences, Boston
University, Boston, Massachusetts

Nicholas A. Ashford, J.D., Ph.D., Senior Research Associate, Center for Policy
Alternatives, Massachusetts Institute of Technology, Cambridge,
Massachusetts

Lee K. Benham, Ph.D., Associate Professor, Department of Economics, Washington University School of Medicine, St. Louis, Missouri

Robert L. Biblo, President, Harvard Community Health Plan, Allston,
Massachusetts

Paul N. Bloom, Ph.D., Assistant Professor of Marketing, University of Maryland, College Park, Maryland

Michael D. Bromberg, Executive Director, Federation of American Hospitals,
Washington, D.C.

Rick J. Carlson, J.D., Mill Valley, California

Arthur G. Carty, President, Blue Cross of Massachusetts, Inc., Boston,
Massachusetts

Morris E. Chafetz, M.D., President, Health Education Foundation, Washington,
D.C.

George R. Dunlop, M.D., Past President, American College of Surgeons, Worcester, Massachusetts

Richard H. Egdahl, M.D., Ph.D., Director, Center for Industry and Health Care, Academic Vice President for Health Affairs, Boston University, Boston, Massachusetts

John Friedland, Research Analyst, Center for Industry and Health Care, Boston University, Boston, Massachusetts

Robert F. Froehlke, President, Health Insurance Association of America, Washington, D.C.

Arthur E. Gass, Industrial Hygenist, Office of Training, Occupational Safety and Health Administration, Washington, D.C.

Paul M. Gertman, M.D., Director, Health Services Research, Boston University School of Medicine, Boston, Massachusetts

Harold Gilbert, Consulting Actuary, George B. Buck Consulting Actuaries, Inc., New York, New York

Willis B. Goldbeck, Executive Director, Washington Business Group on Health, Washington, D.C.

Emlyn I. Griffith, Member, New York State Board of Regents, Rome, New York

C. Rollins Hanlon, M.D., Director, American College of Surgeons, Chicago, Illinois

Clark C. Havighurst, J.D., Professor of Law, Duke Law School, Durham, North Carolina

Geoffrey V. Heller, Executive Vice President, Health Care Federation, University of California, Berkeley, California

David B. Hershenson, Ph.D., Dean, Sargent College of Allied Health Professions, Boston University, Boston, Massachusetts

R. Hopkins Holmberg, Director, Health Care Management, Boston University Graduate School of Management, Boston, Massachusetts

Bruce W. Karrh, M.D., Corporate Medical Director, E. I. DuPont de Nemours, Wilmington, Delaware

Warren Kantrowitz, M.D., Administrator for Ambulatory and Special Care, University Hospital, Boston, Massachusetts

Saul M. Kilstein, Assistant to the Director, Washington Business Group on Health, Washington, D.C.

Elizabeth M. Kurella, Public Relations Associate, Chemical Communications Department, Upjohn Company, Kalamazoo, Michigan

Michael E. Lawson, Ph.D., Associate Dean, School of Management, Boston University, Boston, Massachusetts

Sol Levine, Ph.D., University Professor, Chairman, Sociology Department, Boston University, Boston, Massachusetts

Christopher Lovelock, Associate Professor, Harvard Business School, Boston, Massachusetts

Robert S. Lurie, Senior Director, Systems and Management Analysis, Harvard Community Health Plan, Allston, Massachusetts

Alasdair C. MacIntyre, Ph.D., University Professor, Chairman and Professor of Philosophy, and Professor of Political Science, Boston University, Boston, Massachusetts

John A. McLaren, M.D., Vice President of Marketing, Evanston Hospital, Evanston, Illinois

H. Frank Newman, M.D., Vice President, Kaiser Foundation Health Plan, Inc., Washington, D.C.

Robert D. Reinecke, M.D., Professor and Chairman of Ophthalmology, Albany Medical College, Albany, New York

Russell B. Roth, M.D., Past President, American Medical Association, Erie, Pennsylvania

John I. Sandson, M.D., Dean, School of Medicine, Boston University, Boston, Massachusetts

Robert S. Smith, Ph.D., Associate Professor, School of Industrial and Labor Relations, Cornell University, Ithaca, New York

Ronald Stiff, Ph.D., Associate Professor, Business School, University of Baltimore, Baltimore, Maryland

Linda K. Stokes, J.D., Health Policy Analyst, InterStudy, Excelsior, Minnesota

John N. Tulley, Jr., Consultant for Employee Benefits, John Hancock Mutual Life Insurance Company, Boston, Massachusetts

Claude E. Welch, M.D., Clinical Professor of Surgery, Massachusetts General Hospital, Boston, Massachusetts